Get
Real
G O D
with

by Phillip Fields

Joy,
Bless you,

ACKNOWLEDGMENTS

I THANK MY GOD, THE LORD JESUS CHRIST WHO SAVED me, delivered me, and healed me. I would not be on this planet today if God, my Father, had not sent His Son to atone for my sin and the consequence of my sin. Thank You, Jesus, for becoming a real man and coming to this planet and meeting me in my real suffering. I cherish the thought of spending my life honoring You for all You have done for me. Thank You for believing in me.

I thank my precious wife, Darlena, who is my rock. She has stood the test of time, trials, and tribulations. Darlena, you are faithful and your presence in my transformation made a huge difference. Your willingness to grow with me gives me lots of encouragement and hope. Thank you for standing by me even when I did not deserve it.

I thank my in-laws, who have been like parents to me. I thank you, Glenda, for being bold in your belief in the healing process. Your unwavering desire to see me free has been and still is a source of great inspiration to me. I thank you, Darlon, my father-in-law, for standing with me on the Word of God with tenacity. What a tremendous impact your influence has been. Because you never gave up on me, I never wanted to give up on life.

I thank countless friends and others who stood with me during my crisis and my struggle in learning to surrender. I needed you then, and you stood with me and it made a difference. I must mention that many of you were not sure what to do, but you did something— you prayed, and your prayers made a big difference. I thank all who prayed and reached out to me when I was on my way down.

I will always cherish several men who played a role in my transformation. I honor you, Brent Sharpe, Doug Fears, Vic Bond, Randy Johnson, and Clay McLean.

It is very honorable to make public mention of ministers who have touched us in deep and personal ways. Clay McLean is just such a person. He is one of the truest men of God I know and is responsible for initiating the inner healing process in my life. His life is an example of how God takes those who are wounded in childhood and transforms them, giving them a life full of hope and a heart for healing the abused. I mention his name because he wrote a song regarding the painful memories, and that song summarizes my journey for overcoming the inner wounds of childhood. Ultimately, we look to heaven and sing, as one of his lyrics goes, "All my wounds cry hallelujah." Clay, thank you for being a father to me when I desperately needed a man's embrace.

My special thanks to Jake Jones for rescuing me from the wolves and guiding the process. I also thank Nancy Kanafani for the remarkable job she did in pulling my ideas together and making them flow.

CONTENTS

INTRODUCTION

I N THE JOURNEY OF LIFE, THE PATH FOR SOME PEOPLE seems fluid and flowing, as though it were moving from one place of serenity to another. My life is the opposite. Life has never been easy for me. I have struggled, even with the revelation of God's goodness personified in the real presence of His Son, Jesus Christ. I find that many believers get caught in the same trap. Instead of experiencing a life flowing along smooth, calm waters, these individuals move from one raging storm to the next, barely having enough time to surface for air. Being storm-tossed seems to be the norm, but overcoming and making sense out of the wreckage from the storms is not common.

If you are one of those people who has landed ashore amid the wreckage from your latest battle during one of life's storms, this message is for you. This book is about the uncommon adventure of finding restoration in the pile of debris the storm leaves behind. In these pages, you will read about a real man who lost his way because of the sound of the wind, the force of the rain, and the raging sea that capsized him, but who eventually surfaced to discover health and wholeness. The struggles are real, the pain is deep, but the healing process that flows from these experiences is deeper and more real than anything imaginable.

You may be in some kind of storm right now. Perhaps you are facing a life-threatening disease, a chronic illness that no one can explain or relate to, emotional turmoil that drives you to be and act like somebody you never wanted to be, or a "permissible" self-destruction such as habitual overeating or being addicted to prescription drugs or alcohol. Maybe you are battling hatred for your neighbor because of deep wounds, basic conflicts from your youth that you revisit over and over, confusion about your life in general, or a lack of hope because of the mess you created when you were trying to survive. Or you might be feeling lost and alone because you have not found anyone to talk to about the deeper issues in your life. If one or more of these situations sounds like you, remember, we all are susceptible to falling away from the truth during times when we are submerged in the storms of life, and it can be hard to know how to survive, let alone overcome. What we must keep in mind is, life's storms will either harden us or transform us.

The tests and trials we face present opportunities for growth, but the outcome is dependent upon our submission. To whom will we yield? Either we yield to God and become softened and pliable, or we decide to run life our way, and we live at the mercy of our own abilities and passions. God offers us salvation. He is the One who throws us a lifeline when we are sinking at sea. His salvation plan includes complete rescue—He not only pulls us out of the raging sea, but He teaches us how to sail.

I did not know how far off course my life was. I was a good professional Christian doing all the right things when I got whacked by a storm that almost sank my ship. I became bitter and full of anger about the course of events in my life and was bent on living my way. The enemy of my soul took me captive, and I didn't know how to get free. My ship was sinking . . . and fast.

I needed more than a lifeline; I needed a transformation. I needed to be restored inside and out. My body was broken down because of all the pain and turmoil I was holding within, and my soul was dark. My lamp was dim and my attitude was sour. Yet when I yielded to God, He took me on a path that involved a total makeover. Actually, the work I needed was so extensive that God had to give me a spiritual, mental, emotional, and physical overhaul. The awesome thing about God is that He is faithful. He empowered me to take each and every step, which, in turn, led to a deeper healing and transformation than I ever thought possible.

This total transformation was not easy. I had to face the real issues in my life. No cheap, feel-good gospel would do. I needed to remove the cancerous emotions and spiritual strongholds that were strangling the life out of me. The process was not pretty. Piercing the darkness of my soul was tough work. It required learning to allow the penetrating light of God—His Word—to heal and deliver me.

This message has grown out of my struggle to know the reality of God's redeeming gospel. One thing I will tell you right up front: finding restoration in Christ has required yielding every ounce of my life to God. I am amazed at how He used all my pain and struggles. My life is a testimony of someone who could not get it right, of someone who could not seem to do things the right way, and yet God in His faithfulness continued to come after me and pursue me. God never let go of my hand, even when I wanted to let go of His.

Heading for the Winner's Circle

The journey in this book is about a life transformed from brokenness to wholeness. You will be learning what I learned: how to live *from* God with your whole being centered on Him alone. I came to realize that God did not intend for me to live as some cave dweller, running from the shadows of my struggles. That's not His intention for you either. He desires that we navigate the high seas as valiant sailors, overcoming the rage of the wind and the waves. I am one of His representatives here on earth, a man who has learned to be utterly dependent upon Him, to stand ready for all of life's storms. I now possess a vision of victory and a heart full of confidence that, no matter what I face, I am able to win. That same spirit of triumph and trust is what I hope you will possess by the time you finish reading this book.

If you are buried by life's trials, then you are being held in captivity. The enemy has you in deceit about the corruption in your life. I pray that you will let this message ring with the sound of God's heart and His passion for you and your complete restoration. Take heed to these words and receive them as a divine interruption that could save you from tragedy in life.

I wish someone would have given me the simple and plain truth about the path of destruction I was on, before it drove me to illness. That truth is what I offer you in this message—the opportunity to take a good, hard, deep look at what you really believe and at what and who is really driving the ship that you call a life for Christ. If you discover that your beliefs do not line up with God's core values, then what will you do about it? I hope by the mercy of God that you will take action to change it. God is not to blame for continued failures. It is time to open every door in your life to a fresh change brought about by a just and compassionate God who loves you and wants the best for you.

God is looking for a way to bless you, not punish you. He wants to move in your life. He is waiting to pour His love into the depth of your wounds and transform your cries of pain into shouts of "hallelujah!" The most powerful force of transformation is the love of God. He will be faithful to intervene and provide that lifeline and rescue plan you need. He will lead you to safety, mend your body, and calm your soul. God takes pleasure in restoring you, but you have to receive His love.

Receiving is believing. You cannot make progress in the journey of transformation if you close your heart off to God. Receiving requires yielding and inviting God into the messy parts of your life. Allowing Him to speak into the depth of your depravity begins the healing process and opens the door to restoration.

God sees you in the winner's circle. You belong in the hall of the faithful. The key is learning to see yourself there. God's intention for you will never be realized if you hang onto your broken image of who you are.

How would your life be altered if you thought the same way God thinks with regard to who you are and what your destiny in this world is? If you yielded to His destiny and walked in agreement with Him, you could become a supernatural force of transformation. I'm going to show you how, as we head down this road together. So get ready to get real with God and be transformed!

Let's begin this journey with prayer:

Father, I surrender. I yield to You. I recognize that I am in a mess. My needs are beyond my supply. But I come to You in faith, believing that You can and will restore me. I pray that You will open my eyes to see and my ears to hear the truth about my life. I need Your truth. I need to know what You think about the situation that I am in, and I need Your wisdom to overcome it. Speak to me, heavenly Father, about my life. Bring me direction, for I am lost and overwhelmed. Strengthen my feeble knees and weak limbs. Heal my body and renew my mind that I might know You. Help me, Lord; I desperately need You. I will do whatever You show me and will follow You in the direction You lead. I know You will restore me and transform me. I agree with Your Word about my life. I am Your son/daughter, and I come to You for salvation. In the name of Your Son, Jesus, I pray. Amen.

CHAPTER 1

A Transformed Life: From Brokenness to Wholeness

Coming to the End of Self

I GREW UP IN ONE OF THOSE HOMES WHERE THE FORCES OF anger, violence, and abuse traumatized our lives. My family life was like being caught in a war zone. Complete with emotional casualties and victims, the battles took place on a daily basis. It was dysfunction personified. Despite all that, when I was just a boy, God began to transform my life by His love. There, in a little country church in our rural community, God touched my life. The cool part of this transformation is that we were a bunch of heathens. There were no believers in my family. Our motto was, "Only the strong survive, so you'd better work like there's no tomorrow." Hard work and a hard life is really all we knew—and it was all we expected.

This vain philosophy was the manifestation of a generation of truck drivers and coal miners. But God chose to reach down in the middle of the axel grease and coal dust, and He cleansed my life with the blood of His Son Jesus Christ. At the ripe old age of twelve, grace, God's supernatural implementation of His real love, became my reason for living. God poured out His love on me and gave me a new hope for a brighter tomorrow.

It was this hope and God's love that inspired me to go into ministry; my calling was birthed through my own quest to know His love. I was seeking answers, and God was faithful to pour His Spirit upon me and allow me to begin to heal inwardly from a childhood of deep wounds. Yet transformation is a process, and the foundation of healing that took place in my youth was not enough to deliver me in the hour of anguish that I would go through later in life.

As children, the only hope my brothers and I had was that some day we could grow up and leave. We did. We all left home like soldiers and went our separate ways. We sought security outside the chaos of childhood traumas and chased after experiences that would prevent us from facing the pain of our past.

I had already had the greatest experience of life—receiving Jesus as my Savior—and that is what I pursued with passion. Wearing rose-colored glasses, I blissfully chased after what I thought was the "right" Christian life.

When I first heard the call of God as a young twelve-year-old boy, mature believers told me that I needed to do three things: go to the "right" school, marry the "right" girl, and find the "right" church. So I chased after all three with zeal. Once I left home, I even waited to marry the right girl so that I could dedicate more time to pursuing my calling.

My whole life was dedicated to serving Jesus with all my heart and spreading the gospel through every means possible—street witnessing, mission work, taking care of the poor and widows, working with addicts and the downcast. I served as a pastoral counselor, the dean of a ministry training school, a pastor, a youth pastor, and an outreach pastor. I preached tons of sermons and taught many lessons in schools of all levels. I was in the thick of professional ministry and felt that I had earned the right to be there, having obtained an undergraduate degree in theology, a master's degree in counseling/psychology, and a doctoral degree in organizational leadership.

Our church was a mega church, and I thought it was the "right" church because I was there. We did it all—from conducting worldwide crusades to having top name charismatic ministries networking with us or following after us. We were on the cutting edge of the charismatic, Holy Ghost movement at that time. We saw people healed, delivered, saved, and set free on a regular basis. People came from near and far to get a taste of our exhilarating worship services. We were up and coming and on the wings of revival.

Beyond the walls of the church, I was a family man. I married the "right" girl, and we were committed to becoming the "right" family. Dedicated to living a sincere Christian life, Darlena and I worked hard to develop our marriage through prayer and other biblical principles, along with counsel and support. Later on, the births of our three precious girls were monumental events that we welcomed and prepared for like the good students we had learned to be in our higher educational experiences.

The children were simply blessings from God, and my heart was full of love for them. Darlena and I were determined to make their childhood much better than ours. We just knew we would not make the same mistakes our parents made. We thought that our education, training, and professional experience were all factors that exempted us from the parental flaws of the previous generations.

Family life was about the good things and good experiences, and ours was balanced with a heartfelt commitment to our church and ministry. Church and professional life was a privilege, and we felt honored to be a part of it. I did not have to make myself go to work. Doing ministry was a natural thing for me; ministry was in my blood. Even as a young person, I dreamed of being a pastor and teaching people about God.

My passion was to know my Creator. I wanted God as much as I wanted life. I was in this relationship for eternity. In all sincerity, I felt that I knew Him and walked with Him daily. Prayer and fasting was a way of life to me. I could not get enough of His Word. I studied

and dug deep to find truth. I was a purpose-driven man who understood my identity according to the finished work of the cross. I knew
God's purpose for my life—to know His heart and make it known. I
was clear about my destiny and passionate about my ministry.

The events and experiences in my life were unfolding in an
amazing way. The truth is, my wife and I were blessed. Life was good.
Time was on our side. We were enjoying the bliss of our youthfulness
without calamity and, comparatively speaking, our family and our
lives looked and felt good on the outside.

I am pouring it on thick in describing my life back then because as
you read the rest of my story, you're going to see that at this point we
really lived in a dreamland called "naivety." We did not see the real
issues that were beneath the surface at work in us and our children,
until one day when a breeze blew through the open doors of our
church and rocked our world, changing our lives forever.

The Subtle Wind of Change

Most people in our church did not realize what was happening at
first. It was very subtle, almost unrecognizable, like someone leaving
the window open and the wind blowing a significant document off
the table, but nobody discerning the movement of anything important. The truth is that our church was hit by a major wind of sorts—a
subtle change of doctrine that caused great damage and not only
threatened the core beliefs of our church body but the very foundation of our organization. More importantly, the substance of our
lives and our relationships was fractured by this false "wind," and we
did not even know it for a while.

We hadn't heeded the apostle Peter's warning, "Be sensible and
vigilant, because your adversary the Devil walks about like a roaring
lion, seeking someone he may devour; whom firmly resist in the
faith" (1 Peter 5:8–9), and we suffered the consequences. You see,
the enemy of God, the devil, blew into camp disguised as a new and
improved theology and planted the seed of a new "belief" system
within the heart of our pastor. This false doctrine was laced with the

seduction of unbelief. In one day, this gifted, charismatic, battle-savvy, armed and ready veteran soldier in God's army, who knew how to fight the good fight of faith, became bewildered about the battle and his role in it. Over time, the effect on all of us in the church was devastating—everything we worked for, hoped for, and believed in was destroyed.

The strangest thing about the event was that instead of recognizing there was a visible enemy in the camp and attacking that enemy, we assaulted one another. Lifelong relationships were crumbling all around us, and many of the church leadership, staff, and key volunteers, who knew that there was a spiritual war going on, were getting picked off by the adversary in the process. It seemed as though a presence of darkness had unfolded all around us. Of course, the real enemy, Satan, was bent on corrupting what we had given our lives to—the gospel of Jesus Christ. We knew that we were supposed to be empowered with the Holy Spirit to fight against this darkness and come out triumphant. Yet, somehow we were like sheep being led to slaughter: We had no idea what lay ahead. We just marched in a line because it was the thing to do.

I realize now that anytime the devil is successful in tearing down God's people, the effect is not just on the individual or individuals who lose the battle, but it affects the whole body of Christ. In our case, we allowed the enemy to split our church family. Some sought higher ground, some stood and watched, several grappled for a position, some wandered in the wilderness, some jumped on the judgment bandwagon, some dropped out of the race, a few covered up evil, and others moved on to seek new dreams. But everybody that cared lost something valuable, because we not only lost each other, we lost our testimony as well.

Personally, my reaction to these happenings set in motion a lifestyle I thought was put to rest in my youth. I was hurt, confused, and stunned because the valiant man of God that I adored and respected had fallen away from the true gospel. Having entrusted my life to him as an eighteen-year-old boy, I looked to him as my spiritual father. I admit it, I idolized him. I had put him on a pedestal that no man belongs on. His strength was part of my foundation, and now it was crumbling—and I was enraged about the situation.

Let me make it clear that this is not an indictment against my former pastor nor is it the focus of this book. My focus will be on my reaction to these circumstances, the devastating aftermath, and what I learned that saved my life and my family. My greatest desire now is to help people in devastating circumstances and see their lives transformed by the power of God, as my life was.

For a long time my response to the fall of my pastor and to the aftermath was ungodly and very judgmental. This pervasive attitude weakened my discernment; rage and bitterness dampened my own flame of understanding. My passion for God was replaced with anger for my enemy, but believe it or not, my enemy, in my mind, was not my pastor, my wife, or any other person—it was me. I turned all my disappointment and utter despair into an indictment against myself. I concluded once again that somehow this was all my fault. I had screwed up, and for that matter I was a screw-up—a self-perception and attitude that had developed in me as a child due to my traumatic upbringing. I thought I had overcome all those feelings in my youth, but I found myself swirling in a quagmire of emotions and tormenting thoughts. With all that churning on the inside of me, my power to war against the real enemy was gone. I took myself out of the fight, which opened the door to a full assault of evil.

Headed for Disaster

The same work that captured me was also at work in the spirit realm, dividing and conquering all the members in our church who could not see the real battle. It took us captive by stealing our power to walk in God's love and, in turn, created an onslaught of pain and agony for many, as relationships, dreams, and hopes came crashing down around us. Like dust in the wind, the ministry crumbled and collapsed, stealing from us the most powerful resource we have as believers—our ability to discern good and evil.

The battle became a great struggle for man-made ideals, intellectualism, reasoning, and a work of the flesh. During the combat, many stepped over bleeding bodies (spiritually speaking) to post their theological flags, their brand of theology. The upheaval was like a street fight that we knew was coming—nobody wanted to see it really happen, and it was much worse than could be imagined. And all the while, the deeper work was that our hearts were pricked by the pain of the division. You were either on one side or the other, there was no in-between ground; and there were casualties on both sides. The fact is that people were hurt because the real enemy convinced us that our brothers and sisters were our enemies and they needed to be attacked.

Looking back, I recognize that I played a key role. I was afraid of confronting things because they threatened my security—my paycheck—so I turned my head toward things that I knew were wrong and waited until the end to take a stand for the true gospel.

My heart's desire was that it would all turn out differently, but it seemed like there was no way to bail out the water fast enough from this sinking ship. Eventually the battle became a test of wills. We all felt like David when he refused to confront King Saul in the cave. David said that Saul was still the anointed of the Lord, even though the Spirit of God had departed from Saul for disobedience (1 Sam. 24:6; 16:14), and we felt that way about our pastor. He couldn't be touched or confronted because he was still God's anointed, which made us think that we had no means to resolve the conflict.

The event took me back to my childhood because it was not safe to confront abusive behavior in my home, in the same way we now had no recourse with our pastor. I played the same role in adulthood that I did as a child: I kept my mouth shut because I was afraid of stirring up trouble for myself. The internalization of my pain and frustration was all too familiar and would prove to be nearly fatal. The breeze that blew into our church was now raging in my heart, and it was a defiling experience. Inwardly, I was growing darker and darker, but I was unaware of the condition of my soul.

Soon my disappointment turned into unbelief. I became cynical about everything I valued as truth and everything I held to be true. My thoughts were invaded with a multitude of questions: *Why was the Lord allowing this to happen? Why would God allow people to be hurt so deeply? Whose fault is this mess? Who sinned, the one deceived or those who judged him for being deceived?* Neither I nor anyone else around me had the answers. I became void of any hope for a resolution to my current anguish, and a state of confusion set in.

My conclusion was that we had lost the war, and even more poignant, that I had lost the war. Bitterness, resentment, and anger are dangerous emotions to hold onto, but that's what I did. I couldn't get over the fact that I had sowed some of the most precious years of my life into the "right church," investing in treasured relationships and building a ministry that touched people worldwide, and it all buckled under the influence of this evil wind that blew in one day. I became like a Dead Sea of emotions. All that toxic negativity was flowing into me, and none of it was flowing out of my soul—and I was headed for physical, mental, and emotional disaster.

Another way this devastating event felt very similar to my early years as a child had to do with my fallen pastor. When I was a boy, there was a leader (my dad) whom nobody could stop, even though he was doing things to hurt people. He thought more of himself than he did those whose lives he affected, and I felt powerless to change the course of events. It angered me as a child, and I turned that anger inward on myself; now, as an adult, I faced very familiar circumstances. There were things going on that I could not stop or prevent. I am sure I added to the problem by having an unhealthy attitude about the whole situation.

My worst mistake was becoming self-absorbed. The more I focused on my misery, the more miserable I became. The real damage of this event in my life was how it affected my current belief system. The disappointment turned into unbelief, and I chose to fall away.

Lost on the "Mountain"

Are you starting to get the picture of what my life was like before
I received God's supernatural transformation? Maybe you are able
to relate to something I've shared so far. My life is a testimony of
someone who could not get it right. I could not do things the right
way, and yet God turned my life around. I believe that He wants
to do the same for you. I have more to tell about my past because I
want you to know to what depths I had fallen and what God had to
work on to restore me totally. I am setting the stage to show you how
to find complete restoration in Christ. Only He can turn your life
around and "make all things new" (Rev. 21:5).

One point you're going to learn from my story is that the journey
to restoration and wholeness involves some kind of struggle. In my
case, I was already struggling with the reality of the supernatural
power of God because it was being covered up with a growing pessi-
mism. The enemy did not snatch me away from my first love and my
deep passion for God. I allowed the force of doubt to settle into my
heart and rob me of the abiding presence of my risen Savior. Jesus
never left me (Heb. 13:5), but because of the condition of my heart,
I was no longer aware of His presence. My conversion to Christ had
been radical. Yet the transformation and healing that began to take
place in my childhood wasn't complete, for the process takes time.
Because of that, I focused on my turmoil over the fall of my pastor
instead of focusing on God and His Word, and the subsequent fallout
was like the death of my dreams.

The shallowness of my commitment surfaced. I realize now that
I was committed to my own expectations of success, not to living
for the purpose of advancing the kingdom of God. My ambitions
were driven by the mind of the flesh—I sought reward for my good
behavior, not realizing that I was living like the rest of the world
instead of like someone possessed by the love of God. My early years
with Christ were so simple; I wanted to be in God's will and live out
His call on my life. There was no competition in my heart with the
forces of the world. You could not steal my passion for God away

with a million dollars. I was on fire for the Lord and consumed with a zeal for His presence. However, after the upheaval following the split of my church, my fire was all but out.

I was like the college athlete who spent his whole life fantasizing about playing in the championship game for a national title. When it was my turn to run the ball to the end zone, I tripped, fumbled the ball to the other team, and cost my team the game. I was sitting in the end zone, rehearsing my act of stupidity and the embarrassment of my actions, along with the utter worthlessness of my potential. I not only saw life as interrupted but also bought the devil's lie that my hopes of seeing people transformed by God's power were over. My plans for advancement and glory were like Swiss cheese, a block of substance with holes scattered throughout.

So I did what most victims do—I turned inward and isolated myself from others. I ran away from everything that smelled like church and vowed that I was through with the "organized church." I came to believe that I had failed and was a failure, and internalized that the problems that caused our church to fall were my fault and my problems. Feelings of anxiety swept over me and took me down. I entertained twisted and perverted lies of the enemy that were dormant in my soul: I justified my viewing unholy websites, addiction to junk food, and weekend binges with alcohol as deserved because of the "unfairness" of life. Some would say that unholy sex, excessive food, and stimulating drugs are problems for Christians, and I would agree; but the deeper issue was that I was a naked soldier who had the stench of defeat pouring out of my soul. I had lost a battle and was groveling in my defeat.

The downfall of my former pastor and the consequent crumbling of my church might best be equated to a divorce, the death of a loved one, the loss of health, or some other major life transition. Like many people who find themselves in a situation of this type, I chose to run away from it. We often dive into work or plunge into new relationships, hoping to find relief from the ongoing pain and trauma that ripped out our hearts. Every new opportunity and relationship becomes as a mirage in the desert, a hope that never really materializes, because even when we come upon fresh water, we do not have the capacity to contain it. A healthy heart is like a cup, or a vessel, that has the capacity to hold the love and nurturing of God and others. When the heart is broken, it cannot contain water, or the tender touch of God, which is exactly what it needs in order to receive His restoration. Can you see the enemy's hand in that?

The devastation I felt drove me into a deep state of self-pity. All I could think about was me, me, and me. At this point, nobody could reach me or get through to my heart. I was hurt and I did not plan on showing it. I am a big boy and making my own decisions became my strategy for defense. Allowing someone to touch my pain would be too risky. The only option in my mind was to forge ahead like a snowball hurling downhill. It was not evident to me that I was on a course of self-destruction because I was moving ahead with such speed and velocity.

My embitterment toward the "organized church" made me bent on proving that they were wrong, and I came up with the idea to start a ministry that was the opposite of what I came out of. To me there was nothing more pure than caring for the homeless and hanging out with some real people. I told myself that I was tired of all the phoniness I saw in the church; I would show the spiritually "fat" and compassionately "lean" how the Lord wanted us to live in the twenty-first century. I found myself trying to show that we are responsible to change ourselves because we don't and can't expect the real power of God to intervene on our behalf.

I based this lie on my incomplete experience with church life and my pursuit of God up to that point. I did not see the power of God intervening in the lives of people anymore because I had traded His personal involvement for a high-minded revelation of my suffering and struggles, which I determined were good because they lead to godliness. So I created my own laboratory for pain. My goal was to become a minister of compassion to hurting people, yet secretly I knew that I too was subject to the very bondage that held the street people captive. I traded my innocent dependence upon God for a more forceful, serious approach to life and ministry. I went from living by faith in the supernatural to living according to good works, or at least my best efforts. Looking back, I am not so sure that my efforts or motivations were so good.

A ministry to the homeless fit the protocol. My perception was that if God wasn't moving in the church, maybe there was something stirring out in the world. Little did I know that my running from the church placed me into the hands of Satan. His subtle trap was laid and waiting for me. My whole life was dedicated to helping hurting people. I knew this lifestyle because of the experiences of my childhood; I was drawn to the "nobodies" in society. Yet this homeless-ministry experience felt like a mountain-climbing expedition that went bad. I lost the trail and could not find my way back.

All the while I was walking further and further off the path of God's plan for my life. My intuitive feeling was that I was lost, but I couldn't stop walking; I guess I had too much pride to stop and ask for directions. Subconsciously, I knew I was busted up inside, but I was not going to admit it. Verbalizing my pain was like extracting glass embedded in the foot—I knew it would hurt worse coming out than it did when it went in. So I masked my pain and turned it into "righteous indignation," becoming a crusader for underprivileged, lost souls.

My days and nights were spent trying to figure out how to liberate those who did not want to be set free. The depths of their pain and misery became my new yoke. Many times I felt myself imposing on them what I would not do for myself. I challenged them to deal with the real issues in their lives. My degree in counseling and psychology had taught me how to work other people through their pain, but it had not empowered me to work through my own. Of course, my internal struggles are in no way an indictment against ministers or ministries who care for the homeless and the down and out. Those who care for the poor and lowly are truly heroes in the community of faith, and many of them taught me lessons that will last for a lifetime.

I petitioned God for answers, but heaven was silent. Soon, my prayers became informal accusations at God and complaint sessions about the lost world around me. God was on trial and I was the judge. Why did He allow people to suffer? Why did some seem to have life so easy? Why does He bless some and others He seems to pass over? Why is He silent about the misery of the lost? Deep in my heart I was really asking, *Why are You allowing me to suffer, and why are You so silent?* Yet I don't believe I could have handled the truth if it had hit me between the eyes.

I was not ready to listen to or hear from God. I wanted to soak in my misery. I devoted my spiritual quest to reading about suffering, and I looked for the theme of misery in life. I fed on it. This may sound crude, but I was more at home in the throws of punishment and pain than freedom and victory. I completely lost sight of God's power and the freedom He purchased for us at the cross through grace.

The wind of false doctrine that blew into our church and wreaked destruction in our lives created a vacuum in my life, which caused me to open the door to my past and drove me into carrying this ungodly yoke. Not only was I driven, but my family suffered from the pain of this misery as well.

Cloud of Deception

There's a saying in the world that you always hurt the ones you love. But God's ways are the opposite. He says to all of us to love our neighbor as we love ourselves (Matt. 19:19), and He tells husbands to love our wives the way Jesus loves the church (Eph. 5:25). But my mind was not on the Word; I had allowed myself to fall into worldly thinking, and my wife suffered the brunt of my freshly kindled anger.

I became excessively critical and controlling in our marriage. The lack of fulfillment and the ever-increasing inner pain was reason for me to act ugly toward her. Her inabilities and normal human weakness became magnified in my eyes. Resentment filled my heart because she was hurting and too weak to dive into my newfound devotion for the lost. She wanted resolution to our problems and I wanted justification for my state of inner rage.

Darlena was suffering from postpartum depression after the birth of our second child, and I did not have compassion for her, which is odd considering the depth of empathy that I felt for complete strangers. My thoughts were that I was toughing out my crisis, so why couldn't she do the same thing? She was worn out, but the pitiful sum of my wisdom to her was that if she would just try harder and pray more, then everything would change. My heart was so callous that I could not even see her pain, let alone embrace her and support her. Deeply entrenched selfishness was robbing me of the opportunity to support my wife in her hour of need. The soreness of my soul was like a cloud of deception that covered me and prevented me from engaging with others. My ability to think about anyone else and their pain was impossible unless somehow their struggle allowed me to escape mine.

Darlena's wounds paralleled my own, but neither of us discerned that the same spirit that blew into our church was now in our home. There was division, accusation, resentment, and darkness. We were doing the same thing that we did in the church—instead of fighting the real enemy, we were fighting each other. This cycle of blame and humiliation spiraled into a relationship gridlock for both of us. We knew we were in a jam but did not know how to get out of it. Even worse, neither of us was willing to give up our position so that change and healing could come.

Things came to a head for Darlena when her problems with depression and worthlessness took over her life. It was now affecting our children because she was not able to carry out some of her basic duties as a mother. She was desperate for help and answers, so we took the typical path for help of many Christians—first clergy, then medical. But the medicine, which was for temporary improvement, had a drastic effect on her. This awesome mother and dedicated wife went from being buried under her problems to literally not caring at all about anything (a side effect of the medicine). She was totally out of touch with me, and she was spiraling into the depths of her own self-destruction.

We were both so focused on ourselves that we were unaware of the spiritual battle that was consuming us—a setup for catastrophe. Her remedy for our problems was to check out, and mine was to drive harder with every ounce of energy I could muster. She was busy trying to hide her problems, and I was busy denying them.

With each disappointment, the anger increased, often about stupid things like disagreeing on where to go for dinner. The explosions would turn into days of silence and hours of torment. On top of that, I worked like a Trojan soldier every day with little fruit to show for it. We started a construction business to provide employment opportunities for the men who were seeking help through our ministry, but they worked as long as they wanted something, and then they quit, which made for horrible work performance with local contractors. I was constantly putting out fires and babysitting grown men.

I eventually grew tired of trying to be a Mother Teresa to addicts and alcoholics who only wanted pocket money for their next fix. They were not changing, no matter how compassionate I was. Even more importantly, my so-called crusade to bring correction to the "organized church" was lost in a massive pile of unresolved issues in my heart. It wasn't long before my life came to a screeching halt. I got sick. I burned out and up, and all my bodily systems were consumed.

The darkness in my soul was no longer just emotional problems and spiritual torment; it was disease—I contracted hepatitis B, and I had fibromyalgia pain in my muscles and chronic fatigue. A number of potential diagnoses were considered, but the bottom line was that I was deathly sick. Everything I ate passed through me like water, I had a constant fever, I could not sleep, I was in pain all over my body, and mentally I was in pure torment.

The worst part of the entire calamity was the fear. Fear gripped me night and day. I had no ability to stop the fear from controlling my mind. It seemed like every other thought was dreadful. I spent all of my energy trying to beat back the forces of fear, yet even when I prayed, the dread overpowered any attempt to find peace with God. There was no escape from the fear. Every ache in my body fueled panic, and the panic fueled pain. The two forces were symbiotic; they fed off of each other. The more I worried about being sick, the sicker I became. I could not stop the pain, nor could I heal myself. The entire situation was surreal.

Because all of my faith seemed to have passed away during my self-righteous crusade for justice, I sank into the fear with quiet desperation. The fear literally shut me down. The virus in my body was reflecting the struggle in my soul, but I did not know how to stop either. The virus ate away at the good cells in my blood, and the torment in my soul gnawed away at the security in my heart. I went from being Mr. Invincible to becoming Mr. Passivity. It all seemed like a really bad dream.

My real problem, though, was not my physical infirmity; it was my belief system. Although deep in my heart, I knew the truth— that God could and would restore me—I was in bondage to spiritual corruption based on a man-centered theology that I had picked up and digested. Because of my disappointment with the organized church, I had come to believe that restoration was only for those who were strong enough and educated enough to repair their lives themselves. My belief was simple: God set the world in motion, but if anything good was going to happen to me it was because I charged after it like a shark to the scent of blood.

All the while, deception, the spiritual force of darkness, separated me from being able to receive God's grace, His supernatural power. With the devil as my coach, I separated myself from the goodness of God. My thinking had become so twisted that I put God on trial for abandonment. In my thinking, He was not who He said He was. Little did I know that in order for me to really know Him, my false beliefs needed to be exposed and dethroned.

I reached for faith but could not find it. Every time someone said God would heal me, I desperately wanted the healing—yet I disqualified it with my unbelief. My spirit said, *Maybe that can happen*; but my flesh said, *I don't deserve it*. Instead of believing the voice of my spirit, I sank deeper into desperation. I prayed many foxhole prayers: "God, if You will just get me out of this one, I promise I will serve You without compromise the rest of my life."

Eventually the climax of the pain created an open door for my marriage to fall to an all-time low, and Darlena secretly made plans to leave me.

My ministry was my mistress, and my attitude of control drove Darlena into frivolous cycles of activities and events, seeking fulfillment outside of our relationship. We both carried responsibility in the relationship, but as head of the household and covering for the family, I was failing to provide. I don't blame her for wanting out—deep inside I wanted the same thing. I spent more time wrapped up in my self-pity than I did taking care of the needs of my family. But by the grace of God, Darlena was moved with compassion to help me and stand with me when I became sick. She was and is a lifesaver for me. God used her in many ways to restore me. She never judged me for my failures, nor did she condemn me for my sin. Her support would prove to be the backbone of my healing.

It's Time to Get Real

We got busy looking for answers to my dilemma. We had no income, no insurance, and no options, but what I thought was a recipe for disaster was a very enticing opportunity for God. A man discovers who his true friends are in a crisis, and the church that we attended after the fall of the other one was a breath of fresh air. Many people in the church stepped forward to help us. They represented the voice of grace, which was just what I needed—a supernatural impartation of God's favor. I did not want to admit how wrong my attitude was, and I was embarrassed by my failures—but a lot of church folks came to my aid, despite my struggles. Looking beyond my faults, they saw my needs. That sounds like love to me.

I chose many paths to getting healed and fully restored. The first order of business was to get a clear medical understanding of my affliction. The doctors who helped in the initial process were lifesavers, providing treatment and understanding based on their expertise. But they could only take me so far. Though the treatment I received got me out of the initial crisis, I had in no way won the war. I continued to have pain throughout my body and to experience other complications as well.

At that time, I was a praying machine. While doctors were poking me and checking me out, I was seeking God with all the strength I could muster. I was sleeping about two to four hours a night, so I did not have much ability to focus, and faith eluded me. I would like to say that I was this giant of faith, but I was more like a mouse without resolve. I knew on an intellectual level that God was a healer, but I did not personally have any experience with the process. During the years I had been in ministry, many people around me had received healing, but I was not in touch with it myself. I tried to have faith and do things that seemed full of faith, but all my efforts produced no results. Instead of getting better, I got worse. My conclusion was a familiar one—there was something wrong with me.

I knew deep inside that I was the problem. I figured that if I could not receive healing for myself maybe someone else could have "enough faith" for me, like the man in the Bible whose four friends lowered him through a roof to Jesus, and He said that the faith of his friends made him whole (Mark 2:1–5). So I sought the best men of faith that I knew to pray for me. Yet I experienced the same conclusion that something was wrong; it was not supposed to work this way. Jesus told some of the people He prayed for that their faith had made them whole. Why couldn't I muster up enough faith? What was I doing wrong? I went into deep introspection.

My fear increased because not only was I afraid of dying, I was afraid of judgment from God. I thought that I had gone too far in my fleshly struggles and the illness was a consequence for my bad behavior. I believed I deserved the pain I was experiencing. My despair turned into depression when a friend came to my house and told me that God would give me the strength to "manage my pain." I guessed that if God was punishing me for my sin, then He would give me the strength to endure it. The same tape from my childhood kept running over and over in my head: *This is what you deserve; now endure it.* Self-hatred sank into my heart. I heard the voices of the past screaming at me and hurling insults at me. The words ran through me like a hot iron, and I kept thinking, *This whole mess was my entire fault; I am disqualified from God's grace.* I felt as though there was no hope for a burned-out preacher who knew better.

But God never gave up on me. He was orchestrating my total restoration.

My precious mother-in-law, Glenda Drake, was a key player in helping me get to the root of my problems. She is a deeply spiritual woman who knows how to pray with faith and believe for healing, and she introduced me to a level in the spirit realm that I had long since given up on ever understanding. Her premise was simple: somehow the enemy, Satan, had brought this calamity upon me with my cooperation. She introduced me to ministries and books that helped me understand the spiritual forces behind my disease, and for the first time, things made sense.

Then God spoke to me in my heart and the light came on. His message was pure and simple—it was time to "get real." All this time I was craving the voice of the Lord, and when I finally heard it, it rang true for me. He made it clear that He would heal me, but there was a process of transformation that I needed to go through. The transformation was about getting real and allowing Him to touch me where I was hurting.

The first step was to allow Him to reintroduce me to a deeper work of His grace than I had ever known before. I found out that I serve a very real God. He is so real that He became a man to show me how to overcome the real suffering I was presently subject to. He chose to enter into my suffering long before I was born. The fact is, the Lord Jesus Christ became a real man from the town of Nazareth, entered into my sin-filled world, and made a way for me to be delivered from my very real suffering. (I'll delve into this concept later on.) The depth of that good news was the substance of my healing, but it would come like the drops coming down from an eye-dropper at first.

One of the most important things I discovered in this process was that the key to healing is receiving. It took me a while to learn to receive because I had many issues to work through. In fact, if there was ever a person who had a lot of issues to work through and overcome, I was that person. I was a counselor and minister who needed a lot of counsel and ministry.

The big revelation that began my healing was an old one, but it was reborn within me like fresh oil for a tired soul. Once I started to realize that God's favor was based upon yielding to grace, not deserving it, I started to make progress. Then Darlena and I began searching for some answers to our deep questions, and we found them. The first place we started was taking a long look at the key issues in our lives.

I learned that my sin and the development of spiritual strongholds could prevent me from walking in God's full grace. For instance, God promised to restore me, which is part of the package within His salvation plan, but holding onto my fears that He was judging me would only separate me from Him. If my kids run from me when they do wrong, then there is no way to resolve the issues until we sit down and reason together. I found that I could be sitting in an anointed meeting where there are people getting healed and delivered all around me, but if I am holding onto bitterness toward my brother or sister, I cannot receive from God because I have an obstruction in my own soul. That was another revelation to me—my sin prevented me from receiving what God had already provided, but it did not disqualify me from it.

This became very simple for me. I realized that my struggles and my putting God on trial were fueling unbelief.

The Path to Transformation

Unbelief is like a force field that prevents our receiving from God. I know this from personal experience. Emotions such as anger, bitterness, rejection, and fear were all forces I was carrying around that were defining my beliefs about God, Satan, and me. My whole identity was immersed in my suffering to the point that I came to believe this was my calling, and I was fulfilling my own prophecies. Unbelief was the foundation for all my struggles, and it manifested in anger and resentment toward others. My raging about the suffering of mankind created a no-fly zone between me and God—I could not hear His voice and, consequently, I could not receive His goodness. I disqualified myself with my own unbelief.

The battle was in learning to receive. My thinking was very twisted. I thought that I could not change, and the truth was that I couldn't, certainly not on my own power. That is where I was lost; because I had seen little evidence of God's power in the modern-day church, I was not confident that I could find the power to change, let alone the power to heal. But God is faithful, and that fact is the silver lining of this story.

I was looking for something that already fit my paradigm of thinking. I wanted God's touch, but I wanted it to be non-threatening and ego-boosting. I was asking God to bless my mess, but the Lord had a different plan. Light and dark do not mix, nor does God cohabit with evil. The junk growing in my life was evil. There is no other way to consider it. I now know Jesus defeated the enemy, but at that point I did not, and I was losing a critical battle with him. There was a force of ungodliness within me that made me feel out of control. Deep in my soul I could not stop being angry, bitter, and fearful. I needed help, but I was not sure where to turn.

Somehow I had opened my life up to this torment and I wanted to shut down every door that was open. I previously thought that Christians, especially serious believers, could not be oppressed by the devil, but it is hard to rule out something theologically when you experience it firsthand. The enemy captured the most precious thing I had in my arsenal—my faith in the risen Christ. As a result, my whole belief system was infected with a toxic, lifeless, me-centered, good-works, rational kind of faith. But whether my theology was good or bad, I was dying—and I needed to get to the root of my problems.

I looked high and low for answers; I stood in long healing lines, I called ministries by phone, I went to seminars and meetings, hoping someone would help me shake loose from the devil's grip on my life. Finally, I found help and deliverance. The process was simple, but real. God started delivering me and teaching me how to fight the spiritual battle, and what I learned I have written in this book.

The bottom line is, deliverance worked. I will give you the details in a later chapter, but it worked. Healing came with deliverance. I know that may seem strange, but it transformed my life. I was like one of the ten lepers who, after God cleansed them and healed them, returned to Jesus to thank Him and to glorify God, and Jesus granted him wholeness (Luke 17:11–19 KJV). I wanted wholeness too.

My transformation did not come about because I used certain methods that only a few people are aware of or understand. Rather, my transformation developed out of a simple, pure practice that freed me from bondage. Sin creates strongholds that lead to death. Paul confirms this truth by saying that sin, or the mind of the flesh, is death (Rom. 6:23). This passage does not imply that sin brings instant death, but that sin produces a certain way of life. I was trapped in a way of life supported by thoughts and beliefs that were producing death. It was God's mercy to give me time to work out these issues in my life.

My wife, who was trying to support me, dipped into the same well with me, and she gained freedom from depression, TMJ, and hypoglycemia. She was so transformed that her life took on a new dimension—she became a different person right before my eyes. Our kids even noticed it, and the process made an impact on them too. Darlena was so changed that she did not know how to be the new person she had become. What had once seemed an irremovable weight of depression and heaviness covering her soul was completely gone. The Lord forced the worst issues in her life to the surface, and drove the darkness from her soul with His loving embrace.

I would like to say that we were entirely delivered and all our problems went away, but that is not true. It was more like we rediscovered the power of God, and the Holy Spirit led us on a path that included victory. Each battle opened the door to a greater understanding of the fullness of God's atonement (the offering made for our sins) paid for by the death, burial, and resurrection of Jesus Christ. We deepened our understanding of grace, and the Lord increased our freedom by changing us with His transforming power.

The Healing Journey Begins

The move of God's power is about one thing—conveying His love to His people. The healing journey began when I realized how much the Lord loved me and how much He wanted my transformation for my sake. The love of God is about His substance, and the forgiveness and healing flow are a result of His love. The Lord awakened me to His goodness, which was a balm for my broken heart. He embraced me with grace when I deserved judgment and delivered me from the chains of bondage. This story gets better and better. God never intended for me to get sick. He was trying to lead me away from the grasp of the captor all along. God provided an out on many occasions, but I was blind because my faith was overshadowed with reason.

There were people God sent into my path to warn me. God used my wife, Darlena, but I would not listen to her because of my need to remain in control. I call that stupidity. God puts two people together because it takes two to become one, in God's economy (Matt. 19:5), yet we throw out one because he or she doesn't endorse our crazy thinking. Well, I learned my lesson. Others, longtime friends, pastors, and peers spoke into my life, but it all fell on deaf ears. I was neither reachable nor teachable—the most dangerous posture a believer can take.

I remember an experience that happened one day at a city dump where we unloaded debris for the construction business. I was struggling to unload this mess, and the chain I was using was hung on some garbage. I struggled for what seemed an eternity, and my thinking became futile: *I will never get this stuff unloaded; I'll never get it to become free.* The thoughts were swirling in my head, crushing me down further and further, and I was physically exhausted, when this great big brother stepped down out of a gigantic bulldozer and offered to help me. He freed me when I could not free myself. The chain snapped loose instantly, and he smiled from ear to ear and said he would help anytime. That was the voice of God to me, a lifeline I could not provide for myself, even though I was determined to prove that I could do it myself. Thank God for His grace and mercy.

My healing came gradually and progressively. I did not experience a onetime miracle, but a seed of transformation was planted within my soul that led to restoration. My responsibility was to provide good soil, and God provided the seed—His Word—and He watered it with His Spirit. The power of God transformed me by healing my body and giving me back my zeal for God. I will never forget the last conversation I had with my doctor during this time. She explained to me that my blood was clean and that my body was in good shape. I needed a few minor touch-ups, but that was all. We had become friends, and the transformation in my life had touched her as well. The journey continues to this day, but I was armed again with the power of God and a sound mind.

I am writing this book because my journey has led me to discover that there are thousands of New Testament Christians who are on a similar path. They have known God on a certain level, but they "struggle to get beyond their struggles." Many are sick physically or emotionally, and they are looking for answers. Believers who struggle are meeting in coffee shops at Christian bookstores, at work in break rooms, on the soccer field, or even in the chiropractor's office, seeking answers to their maladies. You may be one of them. I am attempting to give these hungry souls food that does not come from the fast-food, quick answer, Bible bullet hors d'oeuvre table, or something that is not so overcooked that it no longer looks like food. This book is from my heart, and it is real and raw in its attempt to get to the root problems and serve those who need help on a deep level.

I shudder to think of leading anyone astray from a consuming passion for the Lord. He is not our problem, but as you saw in my life, our difficulty lies with our beliefs. Most of us could give text-book answers for many of the problems we face. Yet we cannot seem to gain the fruit of the lofty beliefs to which we attest. That's why I have thrown out most of my "good" and "acceptable" theology in order to find some real answers to the deep issues that I am sharing with you. This book is not a theological treatise on why we do not get healed or why we do get healed. I find that those books diminish faith and exalt reason. I am looking for an opening to ever-increasing faith that leads to mountain-moving transformation.

I invite you to join me on the road to God's transformation. The things I learned on the path of "getting real" saved my life, restored my marriage, and produced a legacy for my children—and I believe they'll do the same kind of work in your life. Joining me means tossing out your good religion for a brand of believing that changes outcomes and produces divine nature in the weak and desperate. Be careful. This book is designed to stir you beyond the walls of garden-variety, normal Christianity. It will at least cause you to question everything that seems so "right."

Before we go further, I appeal to your heart and invite you to answer these questions: Are you held captive? Does the gospel you believe create a synergy of transformation for you and those around you? Would the gospel you believe send Jesus to the cross? The church's beliefs may be doctrinally sound but are, in practice, weak**.** So we're going to begin our journey together by looking at what we believe (ideas we may think are right, but are misconceptions), what we're missing, and where we go from here. Your life may depend on it.

CHAPTER 2

WHAT IS SO WRONG ABOUT OUR "RIGHT" THINKING?

Examining the Reality within the Church

OUR RIGHT THINKING IS JUST THAT—RIGHT THINKING. Our cognitive resolve often remains where it starts—in our heads. The problem with emphasizing getting our act together by getting our thinking right is that we can do it and totally ignore the Spirit of God. This creates bigheaded theology that appears as strength, but in many cases is a setup for a downfall. Wise King Solomon said that pride comes before a fall (Prov. 16:18), which is why the devil wants us to be self-confident (prideful) in our theology. He knows that, ultimately, we can easily be deceived if our own voice is our final vote.

Satan trembles at the thought that we would be consumed with passion for living in the presence of God day and night. Knowledge alone does not intimidate him, nor does it empower us to overcome. Great people—who possess the knowledge of what they should do and how it should be accomplished—are taken down all the time because they lack the power to get the job done.

Peter, the bold apostle, is a great example of one who lacked power. He knew Jesus was the Christ, the Messiah. However, he was deceived by Satan because, for some time, Peter believed that Jesus would establish the kingdom of God by brute force. Peter staked his life on it, at one point rebuked Jesus (Mark 8:32), and later displayed that force by chopping off a man's ear (John 18:10). Yet Jesus spoke to Peter regarding the issue as if he were controlled by Satan himself: Jesus rebuked Peter (Mark 8:33) and soon after told Peter that he would deny the Son of God in the very near future (Mark 14:30). While this account is true, we must remember that when Peter was filled with the Spirit in the Upper Room (Acts 2), he became another man and played his role in establishing the founding of the church. As his story illustrates, the right knowledge alone does not empower us to live as kingdom believers—we need more.

So what is the church missing, what do we need, and where do we go from here?

I believe the "more" that we need comes from being filled with the Spirit of God and learning to walk in His authority and power. Peter's transformation shows us why the church needs the Holy Spirit's empowerment so desperately. Jesus talked to His disciples about the infilling of the Holy Spirit before He went to the cross, saying that when He went away He would send the Comforter, the Spirit of Truth, to us (John 16:7). If Jesus talked about it, it must be something we need.

The Holy Spirit is the third part of the Trinity—the Father, Son, and *Holy Ghost* (1 John 5:7). The Spirit of God is the power of God that can be manifested in our lives when we receive Jesus as our Savior and ask God to fill or baptize us with His Spirit. For the believer, being filled with the Spirit is about being empowered by Him to do and overcome the impossible by adding to us the substance we need to rise above our circumstances. It's also about learning to walk in agreement with the leadership of the Holy Ghost. He leads, we follow. That's been God's plan for mankind all along.

The Bible tells us in Genesis 1:26 that God made us in His image. If that is true (which it is) and God is Spirit (John 4:24), then He would have to make us the same way, having a spirit too. Genesis 2:7 records that God created man from the dust of the ground, breathed into man, and man became a living soul, physically alive. When God breathed into us, He filled us with His Spirit, which made us alive spiritually as well. So right from the beginning God created us with a body, a soul, and a spirit. (See 1 Thess. 5:23.) He designed us to be a three-part being who is spiritually alive through the power of His Spirit and ruled by our spirit, not our flesh. That was how Adam and Eve lived—for a while.

Imagine communicating with God daily, spirit to Spirit, and living an abundant life! That was God's original plan for all of us. Yet Adam and Eve gave this plan up when they committed the first sin (Gen. 3); they died spiritually and their flesh (or soul) became the controlling power in their lives. So now we have a physical body that is governed by our flesh instead of our spirit, and that's where the problem lies.

You see, we were designed to communicate with God and others through our soul and spirit. The soul is composed of the mind, will, and emotions, and our soul facilitates our thoughts, feelings, and actions. Our spirit is the pathway to communicating with God. The body follows the direction given by the soul and the spirit. When we're alive spiritually through the indwelling of the Holy Spirit, our spirit, soul, and body work together to communicate within us to create harmony and ultimately health and well-being. This communication of the vast systems of body, soul, and spirit plays a major role in our spiritual, mental/emotional, and physical health. The spirit leads the soul and the soul leads the body. If that order is reversed, we create problems for ourselves—until we become born again.

The Spirit, Soul, and Body Connection

The body and its complex systems are designed by God to follow a higher order, which is why faith in God is so vital. The body does not have the natural capacity to carry itself. That is the reason Jesus said, "The spirit . . . is willing, but the flesh is weak" (Matt. 26:41), and "You must be born again (John 3:7)—so that we could become spiritually alive and empowered. Bible commentator Adam Clarke put it this way, "Just as Adam was before God breathed the quickening spirit into him, so is every human soul till it receives this inspiration. Nothing is seen, known, discerned, or felt of God, but through this."[1]

The spirit brings us life if we are centered on God. However, if we are separated from God, the spirit is dark and there is no life. Jesus said that the eye is the light or the lamp of the body, and if His light is pouring into us through the work of the spirit, then our body will be healthy. But if we are dark inside, then we will be unhealthy. (See Matt. 6:22–23.)

As you can see, being filled with the Spirit is critical for our quality of life, as it affects the communication between the spirit, soul, and body. A lack of that kind of communication can wreak havoc. Many of the struggles we experience that bring stress in our emotions affect our bodies. Stress produces negative results to the bodily systems. For instance, the heart responds to stress with hardening of the arties, and the immune system is weakened by stress. The stress oftentimes is coming into the body through the soul and spirit. The force of anxiety wears people down and produces many diseases.

The way to overcome this problem is spiritual in nature. So it is important to understand that disease and physical problems are not just random problems. Many times they are produced from emotional and spiritual troubles. This truth saved my life. I was able to work out my physical problems by applying spiritual principles through the grace of God.

The spirit, soul, and body connection is vital. The quality of life that we experience is directly proportional to how we care for our lives. If we are spiritually and emotionally healthy, and we eat right and get proper rest and exercise, then our bodies should be vibrant and full of life. Learning about this connection produces life. Solomon said in Proverbs 3:8 that the Lord's wisdom brings health to our navel and marrow to our bones (kjv). That is life, and an abundant life it is. Yet even though in the beginning God breathed into us and filled us with His Spirit, we lost that connection because of the Fall, the original sin. (See Gen. 3.) When Adam and Eve bought the lies of the devil and ate fruit from the forbidden tree, we became separated from God's Spirit and susceptible to other spirits.

The intent of the Lord is that we be filled with His Spirit and no other. Remember how Jesus told His disciples that upon leaving this planet He would send the Comforter, the Holy Spirit, to dwell in us? (See John 16:7.) Jesus was resurrected, and after His resurrection He appeared to the disciples and breathed on them so that they received the Holy Spirit. (See John 20:22.) This was "a symbol, pledge, and confirmation, of what they were to receive on the day of Pentecost,"[2] when the influence and source of the influence, God's Spirit, came upon them (Acts 2:1–4). They were forever changed by the experience.

The disciples were filled with the Spirit of God and that infilling empowered them to live out the commission of Christ, to carry on the advancement of His kingdom. For example, if the disciples were confronted with a need for healing, they drew from the well of the Holy Spirit within them to speak forth healing. If they needed resources, they prayed through the inspiration of the Holy Spirit to receive an abundant supply that would meet those needs. No matter what the need, they turned to the Holy Spirit to receive power and substance. The church must return to that kind of belief system.

My unprofessional survey of folks that fill up our churches every Sunday morning leads me to conclude that the majority of us act no differently during a major crisis than those who fill up the local malls. We are all searching for fulfillment, and when our lives are squeezed by tough times, we go searching for answers. As church people, we are generally ill-equipped in our ability to overcome adversity for one reason—because of what we believe. My story is a good example of how the body of Christ is typically unprepared for rising above adversity. I thought I was well insulated with a protective understanding of how to thrive in the middle of life's storms. But in reality, my beliefs were no different than the average Joe's. The moment when life as I imagined it came crumbling down, I punched the panic button and landed upside down, wondering what had hit me.

How can such a scenario happen to those who profess to be keepers of the truth? The reason it happens is that our belief system has major holes in it. As I proceed, let me remind you that my heart's desire is not to condemn but to sound an alarm.

No Limitations

Many good and enlightened Christians can explain their brand of theology, but they fall short when demonstrating it. They are a double-minded people; they say one thing and do another. They hold themselves to high standards that are not real to them. The problem is that there is very little power in their gospel. I am not talking about the one we proclaim from the mountaintop, but the one we choose behind closed doors. The one we preach often sounds good, but it does not make a profound difference in our everyday lives. If we are going to make progress as the Lord intended, it is time to make some real assessments of what we truly believe.

It is my understanding that what we truly believe, we will act upon. I'm sure you've heard the old adage "actions speak louder than words." In essence, that's what Jesus was talking about when He made it clear that if we say we are His followers, then there should be a demonstrable difference between us and the rest of the world who claim otherwise. (See John 13:35; 15:9.) Beliefs may include our thoughts, but the substance of our convictions comes down to how we practice what we believe. These demonstrable realities are best described not by ourselves, but by those closest to us. How do our spouse, kids, siblings, peers, and even our enemies describe what we believe? This group of people around us sees our actions and our professions from a different perception than ours.

If you have the courage, ask people close to you what you believe. Then go deeper—ask God what you really believe. He will not hold back. Throughout scripture, God confronted His people with their false beliefs because He loved them. He was not looking to expose them but to empower them. Let's face it; we all go astray. I find that if I am not careful, I just live in my head. I do what I think is "right." Often I find that without the presence of God leading me, I do what is comfortable.

Here is the point. We all get tested by difficult circumstances. The way we handle the trials of life tells the true story about what we believe. If we expect to live life in the footsteps of Jesus Christ, we must be willing to do what He did. Jesus was real, not religious. He made His gospel message plain and simple. He lived what He believed. Jesus did not spend His life trying to conform to the standards of present-day religious ideals; He did the opposite. He exposed the fraudulent foundation of the religious leaders of His day by doing the will of God, not just talking about it. His approach revealed the heart of His Father. Jesus made it clear that God was all about restoring the rightful condition of mankind, which includes deliverance from the consequences of sin.

In His inaugural proclamation from the scroll of Isaiah, Jesus summarized His beliefs about His life. He stated publicly that His purpose for coming to earth was to preach the gospel to the poor, to heal the brokenhearted, to preach deliverance to the captives, recover sight to the blind, to liberate the bruised, and to preach the acceptable year of the Lord (Luke 4:17–19). That is what He said and that is what He did. I do not throw rocks at any church or believer for doing less. However, my life is no longer defined by what I know in my head but by the demonstrable trail of footsteps upon which I tread day by day.

We cannot expect supernatural transformation in our lives unless we do what Jesus did. He gave up His life so that He could become a vessel of absolute demonstration for the sake of the kingdom of God. Every move Jesus made was about doing the will of His Father. Jesus was real in His beliefs because He followed His own teachings with real-life demonstrations. He did not just say it was a good idea to heal people; He did it. He did not just talk about casting evil spirits out of people; He did it. He did not just talk about forgiving people for their sins; He did it. He did not just preach the gospel of salvation; He did it—by demonstrating the gospel of the kingdom of God.

Salvation (the work of His grace) combined with our faith offers us a foundation for relationship with God. Receiving grace to cleanse our sins prepares us to advance in His kingdom, not to "stall out" on the back row of the church while the paid minister does most of the acting on faith.

God's kingdom is about setting up His authority in the earth today. His authority empowers us to do what He did. We have a choice to make about our participation in His kingdom. We either minimize His authority in our lives by living according to our high-minded "right" theology and squeaking out a few good works, or we yield all to Him and become supernatural partakers of His divine nature and vessels of His transforming light. I refuse to be bound by the rational limitations of man—I want it all. I am risking it all to allow God to define my beliefs as I charge after Him as an obedient son. I think the need is to obey Him, not define Him. God is capable of defining Himself.

I know this is radical, but it is real. Many people in our churches are confused because they are seeking the answers to life's difficult questions through logical evaluations and explanations. We must put behind us our self-righteous need to pontificate about how God works and, instead, dedicate ourselves to allowing the fresh wind of His Spirit to blow through our lives. We desperately need to yield to God in this hour in order for His agenda to come forth in our lives.

The reason our beliefs have become false and futile is that we are stuck on ourselves. We are often too busy trying to control life by lowering every situation to our ability to reason through it. I learned a very important lesson in my battle for my life—I am not in control, nor was I created to be in control. The safest and most rewarding place for me to be is in the hands of Almighty God. If I spend my time trying to make everything in life fit together the way I want it to, then I will be limited to my ability. I'll run out of energy really quickly and get bogged down with my weaknesses, which lead to endless failures. I must have the supernatural force of God at work inside me, causing me to triumph—or else it will not happen.

If I base my relationship with God on my definition of who He is, then He will not seem much different than me. However, if I base my relationship with God on His demonstration of who He is, then I will rise above my dull existence and become a Spirit-filled man. I want to be known as that man who believed in no limitations, that man who stood strong in faith as God proved His Word in his life.

Stop Dancing the Dance of Reason

We have to start somewhere. One path, the one established on God's will (His Word) and His ways, leads to transformation, divine power, and demonstrations of the gospel. It begins with looking at our beliefs, which leads to a spiritual awakening if we yield to the flow of the Holy Spirit. We become charged with a fresh taste of God, and our faith is strengthened because we encounter the living God. The other path, the one based on reason, leads us to become self-centered and very philosophical. We get stuck trying to prove our point, which leads to arguments, division, and religion. God proves Himself to each generation; the question is, how we are responding to His proof?

Getting down to the nitty-gritty truth regarding our beliefs forces us in one of two directions: either we cling to God or we try to go the course on our own. I know from personal experience that God is gracious and merciful and looking for a way to bless me, but I've discovered that when I try to live life by my own terms, I mess things up. I very quickly work myself into a place of bondage if I am anything less than completely dependent upon God. So I find I can abandon my high-minded position that I have it all together and seek God with great expectation, or I can continue flirting with self-destruction by living according to my "right" theology.

We all want to be "right," but our need to be right often prevents us from being restored because of how we choose to react to our circumstances. We are too busy trying to get our lives in order when, in reality, our deeper need is to learn to follow God. He brings us into our place of blessing as we submit to Him. Restoration is the plan of salvation for us according to the gospel that Jesus preached. If our lives reflect the evidence of God's restoration, then we know we are headed down the right path. We can say our beliefs are from Him if they bear the scent of His presence. If we are doing what Jesus did and seeing the results He saw, then we are living according to the works of God with the fruit to prove it. However, if we are living under the weight of our problems and life is a mess, God has a plan to help restore us, but we have responsibilities to assume in the process.

Let's face it, the journey to restoration and a life of wholeness is at first appearance clouded with doubt. This is the natural thought process if life has been a series of failures and setbacks. We become conditioned to negative thinking that creates a mental block for positive change. Simply put, if we came from nothing and we never experience any real success, then we are inclined to expect nothing good from life. This is especially true when hardship hits our life. A lifetime of negative mental conditioning triggers the dismal thought, *This is what I deserve.* Then, as if the tragedy itself were not enough, the inner turmoil that comes from the haunting reality of our condition stimulates dark and oppressive thinking about our ultimate destiny. The pressure of tragedy is often earth-shattering when it comes to building a life of security based on what we hold to be true.

This scenario was all too true for me. Illness literally turned my life upside-down, and I began looking at the world from the bottom up. My sickness and the inability to deal with it showed me what I really believed. These deep-seated beliefs were more Satan-centered than Christ-centered. The devil convinced me that I'd gotten what I rightly deserved, and my situation became strangely fitting and very surreal. My physical illness paralleled my inner turmoil. Even though I was in pain, it somehow brought me a nocuous sense of affirmation. The worst part was the mental anguish, which soon became the core of my suffering.

In an effort to block out the mental torment, I read the Bible, which makes many references to complete restoration, including, but not limited to, physical healing. I now know that the Word of God sets the foundation for the validity of heaven being a reality on earth. But, at the time of my suffering, I just did not get it. My belief that I deserved death because of my sin was too entrenched.

I was stuck. I realized that my sowing of wrong beliefs had produced some painful reaping. The fire was raging with a blaze that I could not put out. My beliefs were like straw, and every time I tried to put down the presence of death, it only became stronger. Yet the gospel of Christ said I could be forgiven and healed. I was under the weight of the law of my sin, but His grace, on the other hand, was inviting me to freedom. My big revelation was that I had made a mess, but God had a plan to deliver me from my mess. Though sin had produced a natural reality in my life, there was a greater supernatural reality that through the finished work of Jesus Christ (His life, death, and resurrection), I could overcome the penalty of my sin and sickness. The challenge was learning how to exchange my false belief, which started the fire, with God's truth that His Son Jesus paid a price to empower me to overcome my sin by grace.

I wanted it. The problem was that I had the concept in my head, but not in my heart. I could wax eloquently about how the Lord saved me from the clutches of hell, but I could not stop the powers of hell from controlling my perception of who I was as a person. The shame of my sin kept overriding the truth of the Bible until finally God's Word began to trickle down into my soul. I discovered my mind was fixed on my failure, not on His victory over my sin and its consequences. I was choosing to hang onto the lie that I deserved to be punished for my sin.

Yet the whole gospel message is about the real man Jesus coming down from heaven and taking the place on the cross for me and my sin. I was ruling out God's intervention because I thought that I needed to earn it, and yet no one earns it or deserves it. God's work of restoration in our lives is an act of grace. (See Eph. 2:8–9.) He chooses to rescue us according to His nature and goodness; He loved us first, even while we were sinners (Rom. 5:8). His mercy is granted when we become born again, giving us time to work out the failures in our lives.

When all this upheaval came into my life, I was a seasoned believer of over twenty years. My beliefs were set like concrete. There was no need for evaluation of what I believed because there was no crisis. I was a strong person—previously convinced that I was invincible. I had never been sick before—previously believing that I was somehow immune to such an illness. So I could whip this thing, and I would beat it—me, myself, and I. The old family belief regarding hard work (I can overcome if I just try hard enough) took precedence, and I kept placing the monkey on my own back. However, after exhausting myself, I realized that I could not win the battle on my own, no matter how hard I tried. That is when I learned that receiving must come first; I cannot deliver myself from my own bondage. Here's the way it works: God imparts to me what I need; He gives it to me freely if I ask for it.

I needed to learn to receive God's impartation, the work of His Spirit, within me. Sometimes the Holy Spirit brought conviction (never condemnation) for sin (John 16:8) and other times it was comfort (John 14:16), but overall, the leading of the Spirit was to my benefit. It is foolish for me to dictate to God how He is to meet my needs. He is God and I am not, and that settles it.

I found that in the depths of pain I became very teachable and willing to listen. Now, I cannot get mad at the Lord and put Him on trial if I am unwilling to receive from Him. I must learn to surrender to His authority and yield my suffering to Him. What's in it for me? Upon yielding the control of my life and the current situation to Him, I open myself to receive His nurture. It really comes down to one thing: learning to yield to His leading. I found in the process that God was never trying to control me but to lead me. He wanted to lead me into a safe place of healing and restoration.

My problem was that this dreadful experience struck a very deep core belief within me that I had to be in control of my life because no one else, not even God, could be fully trusted. I came to this conclusion because of the childhood abuse I had experienced in my growing-up years. Upon fleeing my parents' house as a teenager, I remember declaring in my mind that I would never allow anyone to hurt me like that again. I became a self-imposed orphan, and at that moment my life was in my hands. Some twenty years later the belief surfaced again. Would I choose to surrender to God and trust Him, or would I abandon the threat to my insecure front of security, allowing no one to get too close to me? I was completely oblivious to how I was hurting myself by running my own show; honestly, most of us are until we are forced to take a deeper look at the condition of our souls.

Our beliefs are not fireproof if they come from us and our attempt to find the "right" theology based on our own personal convictions. What we believe is like our sinful condition—it must be transformed in order for it to stand the fires of life and prove to be kingdom worthy. How does this change in our belief system happen? Our beliefs are transformed, like our human nature, by experiencing God encounters that totally change us. It does not happen because we dance the dance of reason.

Finding New Life

I spend a great deal of time talking to people with big problems. My first question to them is, "What is God saying to you about your situation?" They often look at me like a dog hearing a high-pitched whistle, turning his head from side to side. They are not confident that God cares, nor do they believe He wants to speak to them in their upheaval. This troubles me.

The reason I am concerned is that believers often feel hopeless when they think they have no lifeline to God in the middle of life's storms. My findings are that many Christians do not experience God's intervention during times of trouble. In fact, the reports I hear speak of how doctors helped them, counselors provided insight, alternative medicine gave them a boost, pastors gave them advice, or a family member or a friend loaned them some money or gave them some wisdom. All of these are worthy sources from which to seek counsel, but what about receiving advice from the greatest Counselor of all, God Himself?

I totally understand the dilemma. I did the same thing. I went to the professionals first. That is not a bad idea when you feel like your insides are falling out. Now, I am not against seeking the help of professionals. The thing to remember is that they give insight based on their skill. Their advice is like my advice: it comes from the ground up. All I can offer another person, if I am just reasoning in my head about their problems, is the knowledge that I gained from my own experiences and training. You could take that knowledge and fill a thimble, maybe. Somehow in our sophistication we have lost the most important source of revelation that we need to exist in life—God's presence and His Word.

I like what Jesus said when He confronted the devil face-to-face. The deceiver tried to get him to turn stones into biscuits because he knew that Jesus was hungry. Who wouldn't be after spending forty days and nights in the wilderness without food? But Jesus refused the morsel of bread and declared that His source was every word that proceeded out of the mouth of His Father (Matt. 4:4). Imagine, no food for forty days, yet Jesus still chose spiritual nourishment over physical substance. I think that is a good example of our problem. We seek professionals because we are very earthly in our existence. Daily, we practice a lifestyle that does not include, nor do we think it needs to include, spiritual nourishment; so when life is turned upside down, we go searching for human wisdom.

Through my own experience, I gained a major insight regarding my pursuit of professional help: Those people could only take me so far because they have limitations just like me. Training and technology are driven by human forces. There is only One who can transform my spirit, soul, and body. His name is Jesus. I thank God for the professionals who assisted me along the way, but I realized that I needed a complete makeover that included spiritual cleansing, renewal of the mind, and healing for the soul and body. There are no doctors who can write that prescription. Jesus did just that when

He hung upon the cross and took upon His body the fullness of my self-imposed, pitiful, victimized, messed up thinking, my toxic emotional state, and my unhealthy, broken-down physical body. The Man from Nazareth created a path to turn around all that was wrong with me.

The awesome thing about God is that He provides. He spoke to me when I came to the end of my good efforts and had gained the advice of the professionals, and His Word became life to me. Now I tell people to do one thing at all cost and above everything else: get the Word of the Lord for your life. Do not allow anyone else to speak above it or beyond it. Let Him speak to you through His Word and in your heart, and He will silence the foolishness of all others. His Word imparts what earthly knowledge cannot—supernatural life. Let Him speak to you, and you will find new life.

Are You Teachable and Reachable?

"Unteachableness" is an epidemic in the body of Christ. This very pervasive attitude, which boldly professes "I know that already," is another problem that prevents believers from receiving from God. I can remember people sharing testimonies of God's healing with me prior to my sickness and their words going in one ear and out the other. I was unaware of my own shallow knowledge of God's real nature. Many church people, including those in leadership, lack sensitivity to the deeper things of God. Jesus explained this condition by saying that we have ears but cannot hear, and we have eyes but cannot see (Matt. 13:13).

Pride and a religious spirit prevent us from learning. A *religious spirit* involves a certain pattern of behavior, rules and regulations, and rituals. We have a way we do things, and we do not want God to mess that up. Religion is created for this reason. It is our attempt to set up and control the movement of God. The problem is that instead of inviting God to dwell within, we build fences that exclude Him. Pride blinds our perception. We stand behind our dogma with great defensiveness, even if it kills us. I know a man who went to his grave refusing to allow anyone to pray for his healing. Such behavior is considered faith in some circles; however, it indicates that we are not open to learning new things that could free us because behind our self-righteousness is a stronghold of fear. We refuse to submit because if we open up and become vulnerable, we lose control. But I have found that the times I avail myself to God, He comes in and does something I could not have done myself.

Have you ever tried to teach your children how to do something and they refused to listen? Their will overrides yours, making it a rather powerless situation. In a situation like this, the only mature reaction is to allow them to do it their way until they realize that you were right all along. Often I wonder if God views our lives in a similar way. He wants very much to teach us and empower us to overcome, but we keep yanking the control out of His hand and demanding to do things our way. He could make us do it His way, but He created us with a free will; He will not force His ways on us.

One day God showed me how He needed to give me what I wanted—to be in control—so that I would learn that I actually could not control things at all. He made it clear that when I was tired of running my own show and was ready to surrender to Him, He would lead me into the place of blessing. What would life be like if He answered all of our prayers with yes? Life would be a mess.

Our unwillingness to listen and learn feeds our depravity, and we become victims of our own self-fulfilling prophecies. The mentality that says *because I am controlling my destiny, I must take full responsibility for my failures* actually leads us further and further away from God's protection and care. When my wife was in college, she went on a mission trip to Africa. One day her group was on safari to see the wild animals and open terrain. She was led away from the group as she stargazed at one of the lush rivers. Soon, she summoned everyone to come and enjoy her novel discovery of the beautiful flowing river. All at once the guide screamed "stop!" in his deep African voice, and he ran to her like a gazelle fleeing a cheetah. The exasperated guide picked her up like a football and carried her up the hill to a safe place. Then he chastised her, revealing the reason for his radical intervention—there were crocodiles in the water that could have "eaten her up with one bite." This story is a good example of how we think that everything looks fine and inviting, yet the divine Guide knows better. If we are not paying attention, we could be setting ourselves up for disaster.

I find that when tragedy strikes, many of us do not know how to respond. We blame someone or something because we often do not know how to make sense of our struggle. Our lack of understanding leads to unbelief. We assign God the responsibility for everything we cannot figure out. Our disappointment drives us *away* from the Lord, leading us *to* misery. We become unreachable; no one can touch us, not even God. Eventually, we give up, and the problem is never resolved, only filed in the bin marked *unbelief.*

The real tragedy is that God wants to meet us in the most horrible and vulnerable moments of life, yet we do not meet Him there because we refuse to listen to Him and learn—and as a result, we develop a callous heart. Pride becomes our defense, when all along, God had hoped to be our shelter.

Remember, we cannot get what we are unwilling to receive. We can attempt to believe, but we will be unsuccessful because we do not know how to receive. We do not receive because we do not believe. The lack of results in our lives sets in motion a vicious cycle of unbelief that produces little resolve of our pain. We put forth much effort with little return—we've got big problems and small answers.

In our cushy society, we do not see our need for dependence on God. Most people in our Western world do not really reach out for God until there is a crisis. Yet this country was formed by a people who had a deep dependence on God as Provider. His intervention was a daily necessity, and they looked to Him for their very survival. Today we have reduced our relationship with God to squeezing a few minutes of "quiet time" with Him into our hectic schedules. But God is not a condiment that we add for an extra bit of flavor—He is the meal.

Unbelief reduces God's power to dependence on human potential. One shocking reality is that even Jesus could only heal a few sick people in His own town because of unbelief (Matt. 13:54–58). Although this passage clearly reveals that unbelief can decimate the flowing power of God, still, unbelief remains a common theme that runs through many churches where the doctrines of men have replaced the manifestation of the power and gifts of the Holy Spirit. To protect their good-hearted religion, these churches exclude large portions of the teachings and the life of Christ. I have heard some ministers of this persuasion say, "Why suggest something good is going to happen when there is a good chance it will not?" The real goal is to protect their image and beliefs and not to enter into the sufferings of others. Jesus penetrated this deception often by healing in radical ways, which challenged the standards of the religious leaders of His day. He healed on the Sabbath, forgave sins, cleansed lepers, and even raised the dead, all of which infuriated the religious right.

Our problems are not an indictment against us; they are invitations to discover the real, raw power of the living God, Jesus Christ. The Lord has not buried the truth or hidden it from us, but He has placed this treasure on the path of life for us. His hope is that we discover Him as we learn to overcome. The supernatural power of Almighty God is available for those of us who will come to the school of Christ and learn to exchange our false, empty thinking with the truth—the substance of God.

Go After What You Need

I hear people throw around a lot of comments regarding our needs in the body of Christ. We have a solid fundamental foundation established within most churches about the core of the gospel: *Jesus is God. He is our Messiah. We know our need for salvation. He is the One who bridges the gap between us and the Father. Jesus takes away our sin.* But the one thing that I see we need is His power. The supernatural power of the Holy Spirit, which Jesus entrusted to His original followers, is, at best, flickering within the body of Christ. My purpose for challenging the issue is not to point fingers but to rally us to go after it.

The real passion of Christ was to die that we might live. He went to the cross to open the door for His followers to have a supernatural life. His death was not just to save us from our sins and give us an eternal home. He died to free us from the bondage of sin and death in this life. His atonement for our sins annihilated the old sacrificial system and gave us the privilege to have a personal relationship with God. The substance of our experience with God produces for us divine encounters that lead to a Spirit-filled existence. That is good news!

No matter what your need, restoration is possible to you if you are willing to receive it. You may be hurting because of an emotional, physical, financial, relational, or an unexplainable crisis. You may be shell-shocked by a recent loss or a family tragedy. But God is not bewildered by your circumstances. He has a plan to restore you. In fact, He will always pursue you with a plan of restoration.

Yes, healing and restoration are possible. They can be our reality. The circumstances surrounding us do matter, but what matters more is that God is poised and ready to meet us. Although the statistics indicate it is not likely and there are many voices crying out against us, God's Word promises and offers all believers His healing and His restoration. We do not hesitate to proclaim that a relationship with Jesus produces salvation and eternal security. Why is it we question God's willingness to meet us in our current mess? Our covenant God provides a clear passageway that always leads to life.

My message has been formed through the ups and downs of my struggle to know the reality of God's redeeming gospel. I'll tell you, finding restoration in Christ has required a total transformation in my life. But the value of what I was required to release during the makeover process does not compare to what I have gained—knowing Him and finding freedom and purpose for life.

Restoration for God's people is always yes from the eyes of Christ, but restoration does not come magically in God's kingdom. It is attached to the formation of a loving and abiding relationship with the Lord. He imparts His goodness to us as we yield to Him. It starts with a seed and grows as we learn to abide in the divine flow of this heavenly bond between God and man. I get to receive all of His goodness if I will surrender my life to His leadership.

Armed with the knowledge of God's goodness, I chase after Him. I pray that His passion for me pours into my soul and blossoms into passion for Him. Remember, He loved us and that is why we love Him (1 John 4:19). His love is all consuming; it even transforms our sinful and dark nature into one that is vibrant and full of light. I want all of God and all He has for me. If you want it all too, it will cost you all—but nothing compares to the life you will receive in return.

The True Nature of God

We need to re-experience the miracles of Christ and other divine supernatural encounters of the real kind. The reason is that His miracles are the centerpiece to understanding the nature of God regarding His desire to restore His children. Some refer to miracles as events in history reflecting a unique message for the people of that era. The belief is that God the Father used Jesus the Son to demonstrate His right to be Messiah with signs and wonders. Yes, this is true; the sheer power of His authority was absolutely real. However, He never indicated that His power was only for a specific group of people in a particular time in history.

The deeper message behind the miracles was a reflection of the true nature of the Father. Christ performed the miracles because He represented the heart of His Father on earth. Jesus also commissioned His disciples to bring His reality to hurting people throughout the land. That invitation includes you and me. His goal was to reveal the Father's heart, which is clearly in favor of complete restoration, simply meaning that He delivers us from our suffering. What Jesus did opened the door for us to possess the richness and the goodness of God.

There is evidence that traces the hand of God restoring His people throughout church history. The last century alone records incredible demonstrations of God's power to heal His people. Even now, in this very hour, the power of the Holy Spirit is moving among His people, healing and delivering them in unexplainable ways. That means the supernatural power of the Holy Spirit is real and alive.

God yearns for the opportunity to pour out His Spirit on all flesh. He knows that the work of His Spirit in the earth is our only hope. Can you imagine the Father setting up His redemptive plan for all of mankind, generation after generation, hoping that after He introduced this plan, we would reduce it to something purely theological? If that were true, then the Son of God came to earth, lived, died, and rose from the grave in vain; and, meanwhile, we are clueless and weak as we watch the devil orchestrate the end times. Not on my watch!

I have stopped defining God on the basis of my own disappointments with the struggles of life. I now ask Him to invade my meager existence and raise me up to be one of His supernatural, wild-eyed, desperate children. I sat for years behind a desk and counseled people about their problems. Some of my "clients" improved and some did not. I preached sermons about how to live and instructed people to dig deeper into their bag of discipline. Though I saw various degrees of success, I cannot say I ever witnessed a bona fide miracle during my rational approach to the deep struggles of life.

Now I go to God for everything. He is my only source. Everything in my life is a matter of prayer, and my prayer life is electric. Sometimes I get so moved by God that I cannot stand; I have to lie on my face. The cry of my heart is, *Bring it on, Lord. Empower me to go deeper and stronger after the things that You are passionate about.* I am not just praying for myself. I am praying for an entire generation: "Let there be a major, life-altering move of God in my generation, Lord. Pour it out. Come, Holy Spirit." I believe God's move is already happening and will continue to happen. There are no other options but to go up. I never want to let my limitations prevent the movement of His Spirit.

The people who experienced miracles during New Testament times were desperate people. I am a desperate man. I no longer rely on what I know in my mind alone; I rely on hearing the voice of God through the Holy Spirit. The power of God and His anointing on my life perpetuate everything supernatural. I have seen more miracles and healings and lives transformed in the last several years of ministry than I did in the previous twenty-plus years. I know people who were chronically ill for over twenty years whom doctors could not help. In this world there was no hope for them—but God healed them and now they are whole. I have watched those bound with depression and mental problems be set completely free. Today, they walk in total liberty and have never succumbed to a spirit of heaviness since. There was no formula at work, just raw, divine power, God's compassion and desire to heal and deliver, and His ability to reach in and change them because He loves them.

Forming a supernatural culture should be the norm within the Christian community. The New Age community boasts of possessing "energy" that heals and transforms people. They say they can do miracles and healings with positive energy. I find this assertion to be a deceptive counterfeit because often the "energy" at work comes with bondage, not freedom. I raise this point because, while we are watering down our gospel to become relevant and politically correct, the deceiver is staging a coup to steal away the souls of men by using smoke and mirrors. Satan is the deceiver who counterfeits the power of God so that he can deceive people. (See 2 Cor. 11:13–15.) Thank God, we have the truth . . . and we have the power to operate according to that truth, if we will launch out in faith.

Discerning Real Light and Real Darkness

Our archrival, the devil, has a battle plan. His strategy is to convince us that the Lord's love for us is not real. The author of deception, Satan plants lies in our minds, hoping they will take root and grow as furiously as wild ivy. He wants to entangle any God-given truth we have, stealing the life from it and causing our power to wither.

Some of the enemy's lies sound like this: "You're not forgiven"; "You don't deserve health or happiness"; "You can't win this battle"; "Your enemies are too great"; "You're a nobody"; "No one cares about you"; and his all-time favorite, "You don't need God." Whatever the lie may be, Satan knows what tempts us and turns us from God—it's his job to know. In order to win the war, the devil must keep unbelievers blind and Christians deceived.

The battle between light and darkness is won or lost on the basis of what we believe—not on our gifts, talents, or human abilities. We are unable to defend ourselves and defeat Satan if we come against him in our own ability or if we believe that, even with Jesus' help, we are no match for the enemy. But if we believe that our God has already defeated Satan through Christ, we win.

You are what you believe. Therefore, be very careful that your adversary does not deceive you into believing his lies. The quality of life you live has everything to do with the spiritual battle you wage through your beliefs. We will look closer at this kind of warfare later on, but one thing you must learn at present is to attribute darkness to its source, Satan. Likewise, you must honor true light as the presence of God (John 8:12). In the heat of battle, I found myself blaming God for darkness—as if my pain were the result of friendly fire—when, in fact, the enemy was the root of the problem right from the start. The devil is the accuser; he is a master at planting accusations in our minds. If we take up his cause by coming against God or others, we become his slave. Darkness takes root in our hearts and minds, we live under the stress of his lies, and we end up fighting in battle against the very hand that could save us and help us find freedom from bondage and suffering.

God is good. There's no question or doubt that His nature is pure and His motivation is holy. Yet for some reason we blame Him for our deception. We get hoodwinked into believing that God is the source of our problems, and then we fight against Him or we don't fight at all. What we need to do is to break out of our wrong thinking, come out from under this cloud of deception, and see the truth: *God wants us free. He is good. If we will yield to Him, we will find the path of salvation.*

If we want the blessings of God, then we must submit ourselves to Him. It is really quite simple. Through grace, God seeks to provide for us and then equips us to live a lifestyle of wholeness. On the other hand, through manipulation, the enemy seeks to penetrate our life

with evil and then provides a life of torment and ultimate destruction. Since we are predisposed to sin, we are definitively caught in a
battle for our lives. Either we remove the blinders of Satan ourselves,
or we ask for help. But either way, we must get real about it!

God has a search and rescue plan for those of us who know we
are lost at sea. He is just waiting to spot our SOS signal. When He
sees it, He will come on the scene like a Green Beret to free us from
the war within our soul. He desires to set us free, for we are the
remnant, the overcomers who are representatives for our generation
(Rom. 11:5). Our responsibility is to stretch out our hand and grab
onto the rescue rope that our Savior extends. The Father is seeking
those of us who will trust Him like our lives depend on it—because
they do.

Unity Brings Power

Here's another problem of deception we face: There is way too much
competition within the body of Christ. We put too much emphasis on
building *our* kingdoms instead of building *the* kingdom. As a result,
we are divided. We cannot come together for the common cause of
advancing the gospel without arguing over the small stuff. Our arguments usually come down to one thing—who gets to be in charge.

We are playing church. We spend more time vying for position
and complaining that our needs are going unmet than we do laying
our lives before God. Consequently, we spend our time going to
church without experiencing the vital life force of the church. It is
time to grow up—to get over our petty, self-centered, thumb-sucking
behavior, stop hiring "babysitters" to watch the "babies" (in Christ),
and get real in our pursuit of the living God. (See 1 Cor. 3:1–7.) If
maturity is our goal, we must drop the need for control and emphasize what's important: the unity of our hearts, our lives, and our
resources as we focus all our passion on our Lord and Savior.

Think about it like this. If by chance a foreign country were to
invade this great nation tomorrow (God forbid), we would rally
together to defeat it. If strangers were sneaky and hid in places across

the country to terrorize us with surprise attacks, we would work together to root them out. Maybe some would fight with different weapons and/or and tactics, but the common theme would be to eradicate the enemy and restore our country to its sovereignty. We would not rest until we had won the battle, nor would we fight against one another. The only requirement for joining the effort would be to remain loyal to America.

The same need exists within the body of Christ. We have a known enemy whose name is Satan. He sneaked beyond the border security and weaved his way into our fellowships. Now we must unite ourselves to rid him from within and rally for the advancement of God's sovereignty in our communities of faith. The power we forfeit by continuing to "play church" is astronomical. Our complacency and passivity are causing a hindrance to the current move of the Spirit of God and His power among us. The early church stuck together and fought for each other to the finish. God showed up for them in their unity (Acts 4:24–35), and they were known as people who turned the world upside down (Acts 17:6). Let it be the same with our generation.

Let's abandon our formal structures and petty concerns and get after the real business of the bride of Christ. As a married man, if I want passion in my relationship with my wife, I need to pursue her—not just to get her to say I do, but to continue to go after her. I feel like too often after we get saved and say I do to Christ, we get fat and lazy about our pursuit of God. The passion is gone. I am not talking about forms and expressions, but about what is at the heart of our relationship with God. It is time to get radical, get upset, get fired up—to get *something* besides content with the same old boring religion that watches people fade into eternity.

I do not believe we can become too radical. My passion for God grows daily. I am no longer content to be a professional Christian. I am a man who once walked the planet as a dead man, and now I am alive unto God and filled with His power (Rom. 6:11). When I wake up each morning, I believe that the devil and his demons say, "Watch out, he's on the loose!"

The lack of power and authority in the lives of many believers is a problem that diminishes the manifestation of God's deliverance for His people. Folks who are dying (spiritually) walk through the front doors of churches every week, wide-eyed and seeking answers. It is time for us as the church to know we are equipped to minister to the deepest needs within our communities.

The miraculous acts and powerful demonstrations of God have become a thing of the past for many churches. It's as if they have made the supernatural nature of God confidential information that must not be leaked to people within the congregation for fear that someone might be offended and leave the church. This issue is causing many to fall by the wayside, to give up their belief that the Christian church has any real answers for humanity's suffering.

I feel that God is raising up a network of believers who simply want to see Him work among His people. They are not interested in building glittering palaces that serve as shrines to the mighty men of God. They are no longer satisfied with Sunday morning services that intend to appease and entertain. The people who are hungry for God are those who want Him and Him alone. No more politics, parties, and games about church matters and church business. Their attitude is, "Show me God. Teach me how to live the victorious life that equips me to obtain my spiritual heritage in Christ." This hunger to know God and to see Him work is why the remnant cries out to God to bring restoration of His authority and power to the church.

Getting Real about Sin

It has become highly unpopular in many churches to address sin. The term has been euphemistically replaced with words like *issues, problems, faults,* or something soft like *struggles.* Remember what happened to Adam and Eve in the garden after they sinned? God had to remove them from His presence. He still loved them, but He cannot tolerate the sins of man because He is perfect and holy. So when we commit a sin, it separates us from His presence. Many churches have stopped teaching this message because it might be too offensive to listeners.

Get real! What happened to conviction? (See John 16:8.) There are and will be consequences for our sin. It's biblical. This is why our lives become a mess. We create disaster and wonder where God is. Be reminded that He is waiting for us at the cross.

Now, I am not saying we never sin after we become born again. We would not need a Savior if that were true. We are human, and ever since Adam and Eve fell in the garden, people have been born into this world with a sin nature (1 John 1:8). But once we become born again, sin no longer has the reigning position in our life. When we do sin, we can ask God to forgive us and the Bible says that the blood of His Son Jesus cleanses us from all sin (vv. 7, 9). My point is, the church that does not rightly preach the Word of God on sin will not empower people to overcome it.

Churches seem to take one of two stands when addressing sin. It is either the all-consuming evil nature of mankind, which is barely redeemable, or it is the mushy awkwardness of the politically incorrect issues of life that must be tolerated and embraced. One side pounds with the law; the other side fluffs up people with exaggerated grace. Neither approach sets the captives free.

Many claim the need for balance. I agree, but I believe the level of emphasis on the core sin issues should be regulated by the example given by Christ. He embraced sinners and confronted the religious. I believe that translates into a straightforward pattern. Sin separates us from God and that is the issue. Sin should be eliminated because God did not create us to live apart from Him or each other. Purging sin from our lives leads to unity with God and others, and peace within ourselves. But in the process of working through our sin or helping someone else work through theirs, we must be careful to take a humble approach in appropriating God's grace, steering clear of all religious pride.

Do not discount or forget that the Father sent His Son to be crucified and punished for our sins so that we could be forgiven and set free from the snares of evil. His goal was to deliver us from the power of sin, not beat us over the head with it. We cannot be unshackled from sin's power until we recognize that we willingly became a slave.

Cheap grace will not free us. Balanced morality is no real source of power. Our only hope is the nail-scared hands of a risen Lord. We must always keep in mind that receiving from God His mercy, grace, and love, in the real person of Christ, empowers us to live free from sin. Let's look at two key sin patterns I see in the body of Christ that strangle us.

The first sin pattern is our striving lifestyles. We create stress in our lives because we resist the grace of God. He provides everything for us through a work of grace; that is the reason Jesus became flesh. As a man He prepared the way for us to overcome our sinful nature by proving that a supernatural life is possible. When we choose to follow Jesus, He empowers us to overcome as we yield to His grace. Remember, Jesus said following Him was like putting on a yoke, but His yoke is easy, or greasy, as I like to say. (See Matt. 11:29–30.) If we pull against His yoke, we stress ourselves out, but if we yield to it, we slide through life's challenges. It all goes back to surrendering control.

Striving stems from the fear of losing control of our lives. Many in the business world seem to have an insatiable appetite to create wealth. Secretly, they strive to gain influence so that they can drown out their fears of failure. Even stay-at-home moms who seek to create and maintain a family atmosphere can live under this "striving mentality" if they are not careful. Striving affects us all, and knows no limitations of age, race, or economics—but it is sure to leave in its pathway fear, stress, and anxiety. Constant pressures such as these leave our bodies in an unending, low-grade fight-or-flight state. You saw what striving did to me.

This stressful, striving lifestyle sets us up for sickness, failure, and a host of other struggles. We are stressed because we are disobedient, and we resist grace; but God invites us to the cross to change us so that we are no longer self-reliant, independent beings. At the cross we die to self (yield all of ourselves to Jesus) and gain a new Spirit-filled life in return. I have found that until we decide that we no longer need to have all the world can offer, we will continue to be stressed. I almost died before I realized I could not maintain my high-performance lifestyle. I was fighting against the grace of God.

That way of life was not the will of God for me—and it isn't His will for you. I learned the hard way that many of our problems can be solved by yielding.

It is interesting to note that after we become ill—whether the sickness is something simple like the common cold, emotionally tormenting depression, or a life-threatening illness—we often continue striving, seeking cures and quick fixes to get well. In our efforts to heal, we are usually willing to try many remedies. Some people become so desperate to find a cure that they will try anything, without conviction as to whether or not it is biblical. Doing so innocently gets some of them into occult practices. We can avoid getting into error by learning to hear God's voice in our hearts and yielding to His Word.

I'll let you in on another secret that is hidden somewhere behind the pristine pillars and shimmering windows of many of America's churches—self-determination is marketed as faith. Most of us are used to getting things done because of hard work. In our society "only the strong survive," and here in the U.S. *survival* implies "gaining success and status." This strategy may work for a time, in the business world, for example, but it is impossible to carry out when you cannot get out of bed and are too weak to do anything for yourself. After three months in this invalid state, my inflated self-determination had deflated to despair—a place where God could finally reach me. That's how I learned that faith begins with receiving revelation, not by a show of force.

The end to striving seems to only come when life's circumstances force us to face reality. The inevitable happens when we hit a wall—it stops us in our tracks. The wall represents a misfortune of some type. I have found in most cases there are warning signs revealing that a pitfall is ahead. If you see yourself here, I urge you to consider that there is a better way to deal with this hectic cycle. Stop, drop, and roll in a new direction. Give yourself the gift of life; slow down and enjoy the blessings God has given you. I wish I had a quarter for every time I have heard the phrase, "I just don't understand why this (crisis) is happening to me." We cannot see it because we don't want to see it.

We have created for ourselves a false foundation that cannot stand the storms of life.

The second sin pattern that I see within the body of Christ is hypocrisy. This is a scary thing. I've heard people say that sermons on Sunday morning pronouncing our freedom and deliverance are more like wishful thinking than real experience. We advocate relief in various abstract ways without the experience and the knowledge of how to lead people there. We cannot lead where we have not been ourselves. The Promised Land is described in great detail in the Bible, yet wilderness living is the common course for many folks within the church.

God is portrayed as powerless because of our double standards. Hypocrisy is very destructive to the body of Christ because it causes wounded believers to drop out of the church scene altogether. I find that people are not tired of God; they are worn out with religion and its practices. Some people who are hurting cannot find what they need because they are forced to jump through hoops to get answers.

I believe it is time for cleaning house. We cannot expect God's visitation if we are going to live by double standards. When we live that way, we actually condemn ourselves because we refuse to walk in the light. I believe the only solution is to follow the example of Nehemiah and those who were rebuilding the wall around the city of God. Initially, Nehemiah stood, openly repented, and prayed publicly for hours, dealing with their (Israel's) sin (Neh. 1). Public repentance is a measure that will bring humility to leadership and restore trust to followers.

True repentance starts with the heads of leadership. Fathers must lead the way in their families. Pastors and priests must lead the way in their churches. Mayors must lead the way in their cities. Individual leaders must submit themselves to the process they declare to be righteous, the right path. Chiefs cannot say to their followers, "This is what we should do," and not do it themselves. It is like doctors who prescribe a protocol for others but refuse to practice their own advice. Paul said himself that he beat his body into submission so that he would not be disqualified from the commitment to the faith he taught others to follow. (See 1 Cor. 9:27.)

I lead the charge in this area. I repent for my sinful behavior that caused or causes others to stumble. I was wrong, and I am sorry. Please forgive me as a pastor and a counselor who blew it. My testimony crumbled as I walked away from the gospel. I denied the power of God to save and deliver. Please forgive me. I am committed now to being a vessel of His restoration to the body of Christ. I will stand up for the broken and other captives held in bondage. Come one, come all who are weary and heavy because of the burdens of religion: find rest in the grace of God—the real demonstration of His goodness.

A Full-Throttle Encounter

It is my desire that you come away from reading this book with a great passion for the living God. That's what you need to receive all of His goodness and benefits—to absorb, experience, and act on God's living Word for yourself. (See John 1:1, 14.) Now is the time, today, to run after God with all your heart. Don't wait until it makes sense. The bottom line is that until you experience a full-throttle encounter with Him, you will not be spiritually alive. Until His life is overflowing you and drenching those around you, your faith will be powerless. You may be in a lifeless condition because of sickness, pain, suffering, or some other tragedy; but until you leap into His arms, you will not find His safety net. He has a plan for your recovery, *if* you are willing to receive it and obey Him—whatever the cost.

So to know God's plan of restoration for our lives, we must submit to Him. When we surrender to the Lord, we learn His nature. He is good, gentle, and merciful. These are the attributes of a loving Father who wants us to live *from* Him, not just *for* Him. God is looking for real people who want to share His life. The first step to living from God is learning to *receive* from Him; it's the basis for being transformed.

God intended for us to live according to His nature. We are able to do so if we live from Him. Otherwise, we end up dancing in circles trying to get our performance just right in order to gain His approval. Wouldn't it be strange if your child performed for you every day, seeking your approval and each time asking, "Now do you love me?" I want my children to understand that they already have my approval and that there is no performance necessary for me to love them. The same principle applies in our relationship with God.

We are His children and already possess the unconditional love of our heavenly Father by birthright, not performance. We have God's approval, no questions asked, *if* we receive it and apply the blessing of His Son's atonement (Christ reconciling us to God by going to the cross for our sins).

Receiving is the key to believing. How do we receive from God? First and foremost, we become childlike. I did not say childish; that only promotes self-centeredness. Becoming childlike involves innocence and trust. If we expect to receive the touch of God in our life, we must exercise complete trust and innocence. When my children come to me because they have needs, they don't have to reason whether or not I will help them. They trust that I will be there for them. It is a deep and rich truth knowing God as Father and that He has the best of intentions for you, because He knows what is best for you. With that understanding, you can approach Him expecting good things. Expectation is the beginning of the receiving process.

I could not receive from God when I got sick because I was not listening to Him. Truthfully, I was not listening because I thought my ways were better than His. I had the answers to my questions. I knew who I was, and I was determined to pursue life on my terms. Listening required me to slow down, but there was no time to slow down and pay attention to road signs, let alone ask for directions. If we are going to live victoriously, in health and on purpose, then we must be able to hear our heavenly Father's voice in our hearts.

Jesus said, "My sheep [that's us] hear my voice" (John 10:27). Maybe our struggle is that we don't know how to be sheep. It starts with dependence. Sheep are completely dependent upon the shepherd for everything. That's how we should depend on our "Good Shepherd" (vv. 11, 14). When we're confronted with adversity or temptation of any type, we need to get God's Word regarding our specific situation. After hearing God speak to us regarding our struggle, we need to allow His Word to become real to us by acting on it. But we must be sure to wait for His cues and respond in obedience. If we were on a jungle safari and our guide told us which direction to take, we would not contest him, because he knows the way. The same is true of Jesus. He is the way (John 14:6), the map that leads to the promises of God. Learn to follow Him completely.

I admit I was clueless when it came to knowing how to receive when I got sick. I knew how to give orders, work like a dog, and handle multiple crises at once. I danced to the tune of high performance music for so long, it became normal to me. This living *for* God was a mentality in which I carefully cultivated my theology and backed it with impressive performances. I could witness on the streets, travel to foreign nations as a missionary, and counsel the hurting, but I struggled to receive from God for myself. I was armed with information about God. I knew His ways. I even knew He loved me. But my core belief was that I had to fix things down here for Him. I lived life according to a myth, believing that I was doing good in His name. So I learned all the best methods and charged forward, doing everything at my best *for* Him. I was a God-imitator in the wrong sense.

God's plan for us is actually the opposite. He imparts life to us. He gives us breath to breathe. He is our substance. He is our Father, and we are His sons and daughters. He wants us to draw from His life-giving well as His children, not as workers in His field. Daily, we go to Him to obtain new life.

So why is it so important to be able to receive from God? Our whole life depends on it—that's why. It is vital that we learn our place in the kingdom of God, a place of dependence and submission. There is something very real that happens physiologically in our body, soul, and spirit when we rebel against God's model and attempt to live without Him. If we do not, cannot, or will not receive from God, then our alternative is a life driven by reward and punishment.

Ultimately, we must yield to God. Like the man trapped on an island, desperate to get off, we must surrender to the rescuer and let Him take us to safety. The first step involves listening. I am talking about paying attention with great expectation. Modern culture communicates information through a series of sound bites. Listening, in the biblical sense, refers to yielding to the Master and ultimately becoming willing to obey Him. I learned that, in order to receive, I must listen, wait, obey, and stand. This active process propels me into a position of hearing from God. Hearing and applying God's Word is a dynamic process that we will be talking about throughout this book.

So where do we go from here? If you are struggling and cannot get out of the hole you dug for yourself, my admonition to you is to look deeper. No, not at the bottom of the pit you dug, but up above your sin and your struggles where there is a wave of God's goodness taking place right now. God is making ready a people who hunger after Him with all their heart. He is coming after us, not to take us out of this world but to prepare us to take it over.

God's plan is that we come out among the living and lay hold of what He sent His Son to die on the cross for—life, and life abundant (John 10:10b). Victorious living is the essence of being transformed, not so we can be fat and happy, but that we might live a life that extols His goodness and wondrous power, a life that leads to our gain and His glory.

We need to keep in mind that this life is a practice run for eternity. The Lord's Prayer says, "Your kingdom come, Your will be done, on earth as it is in Heaven" (Matt. 6:10). How we choose to flow with God's plan now prepares us for our eternal future. My prayer for you is that you would be so inspired by this revelation that it would stop the cycle of insanity in your life—doing the same things over and over expecting to get different results—and that you would get real, get healed, and get transformed!

Prayer:

Father, I seek You and cry out to You for healing for my body and peace in my soul. I ask You to teach me how to receive Your provision for my body and my life. Help me, Lord, to daily surrender to You all of the heaviness and pain I experience because of my suffering. You are my only hope. There is none greater than You. I cannot go another day without connecting with You. Help me to hear Your voice, to know Your purpose, and to walk in Your light. I repent for running my own show and lay down my will in exchange for Yours. Pour out Your mercy and love, and I will receive it and apply it to my life. Thank You for providing everything for my life that I need to be restored. I believe Your Word, and I trust in Your promises. In Jesus' name I pray. Amen.

CHAPTER 3

YOU ARE WHAT YOU BELIEVE, PART 1

The Driving Force of the Transformation Process

THERE COMES A TIME WHEN WE MUST FACE THE PERSON in the mirror—I face me and you face you—and ask, "What is my life all about?" Until we go through the process of facing how we show up in life, we cannot move forward in God's kingdom. Jesus made it very clear to His disciples that if they were going to come after Him, they must deny themselves, take up their cross, and follow Him (Mark 8:34). Denying self is the greatest barrier to overcoming victory that any believer will encounter.

Our path and walk with God is about exchanging our will with His. God's will is so much greater than ours. Facing the truth about what we believe is like holding our will under an X-ray light and the Lord's will under the same light. Upon examination of the two, it is clear that what the Lord wants and what we want are two different things. We want to be in control and create our own destiny; He wants to transform us and use that transformation as a means to create His glory on earth and for eternity. This concept of glory is something I struggled with for years.

I wrestled with it because every time I looked in the mirror, I did not see the glory of God; I saw my obvious flaws and shortcomings. My image revealed what I really believed; my perception was as deep as my true beliefs, and I would think, *How in the world could that man in the mirror do or be anything representing the glory of God?* I could not go any deeper because I believed I was unworthy of God's glory. But as He began to transform my life, when I stared at myself in the mirror, I saw something different. I saw myself, but in a different reflection—I began to see His image, the image of God, reflecting through me. It startled me to think that I bore His image, that my life now had His imprint. I studied my reflection further and to my surprise there was glory; God's presence was on me. That caused me to realize that I was a real representation of His glory.

It was so much harder to believe that I had His image and therefore reflected His glory than it was to believe that I was a nobody, just thankful to hang out with some good church folk. The basic difference between believers who experience transformation and those who do not is our reflection. I reflect what I believe. If I believe I am a "slave" and I am grateful to have a job and a mere morsel of bread from the Master, then I will live as if I deserve the sufferings of life. But if I come to believe that I am a son who has been granted the privilege of dwelling in the Father's house, then my suffering will reproduce the glory of my Father in all I do.

The foundation of all your beliefs comes from your relationships. Finding out what you personally believe about God, Satan, self, and others is very important on the journey to finding restoration. Discovering these beliefs will assist you in pinpointing what is hurting and what is helping the process of transformation in your life. So in these next two chapters, we're going to continue to look at what we believe. But be prepared—knowing what you believe may come as a shock to you. In my case, I thought I believed in God in ways that I discovered I did not. For instance, I thought I believed in

God's power to heal. I found out that what I believed was that divine healing was a good thought, but I didn't practice it.

When I didn't receive my healing, I was stuck. I didn't recognize that part of God's healing process includes my personal responsibility for the layers of sin that prevented my receiving from Him. In other words, it was inappropriate for me to expect God to remove illness miraculously without requiring me to make some changes. I knew that my driven lifestyle was causing problems, but I was in denial about how it was affecting my health. Learning what I really believed saved my life.

I discovered in life that what you believe you will become. It's like the old saying, "You are what you eat." This instinctive desire to believe is the driving force of our lives. The motivation to believe in something or somebody is common to all people. The formation of our beliefs comes from what we learn as we are working through the experiences of our lives. Along the way we discover by experience there are certain ways that are more rewarding than others in getting our needs met. These confirmations reinforce our understanding and, in turn, form our beliefs.

A *belief* is the firm persuasion that we rely on to have our needs met. A *belief system* is our way of living, based on our attitudes, agreements, experiences, judgments, expectations, vows, and oaths. Our beliefs become real to us as we act on them. In this way, we learn and unlearn patterns as we seek to find a fulfilling life.

All beliefs are motivated by the innate desire to become fruitful. We all want our lives to be full of meaning and substance; we want to be somebody. However, we learn on the road of life that we have limitations because of our human weakness. It is in this learning process that some people discover a need for God. We come to realize that if we are going to live above our human weaknesses, we must learn to depend on God's help to do it. God offers us the opportunity to exchange our human potential with our divine purpose. We each have a divine purpose in the unfolding of creation and eternity. Learning to live on purpose rather than being subject to human potential is the higher calling in life. Living a purposeful life is learning to be the person God called us to be, quite a difference from living just to get our basic needs met.

When our lives are producing less than our divine purpose, it is because we are missing the power of God. Partaking of His divine nature and living above the normal frailties of humanity does not just happen. There is a definite process that must take place. It starts with an encounter with God. He introduces us to a deeper reality, the reality of His Spirit. The invitation to know the Holy Spirit leads to a relationship, and the relationship leads to transformation. This transformation produces a change in the way we see and understand life. We become vessels of the life of God flowing through us, which is like electricity—ultimately, our relationship with God produces power to become His glorious sons and daughters.

The concept of transformation presents a problem for many of us because it is not what we experience in life. In fact, we live a life that is something altogether different. We race to keep up with life's demands and hope that we can squeeze some fulfillment out of our mere mortal existence. A sub par experience is the common Christian life. Let me put it this way: I once heard someone say there is way too much potential buried in graveyards.

If we plan to live as image bearers of God's light, then we are required to allow our beliefs to be transformed by His power. We must allow Him to take us through a deeper change. To benefit from intimacy with God—regularly spending time with Him in intimate, two-way communication—we are called to learn to yield everything to Him. He wants to get to the core, the heart of what makes us tick.

I must admit that going deeper spiritually is a challenge. We are tested because of the spiritual battle that takes place in everyday life. We will take a closer look at spiritual warfare in a later chapter, but for now, we must remember that the battle is between our will, which the adversary uses to deceive us, and the will of the Father. Either we yield to God and produce fruit that proves our surrender, or we control things according to our will, get caught in the web of Satan, and produce the works of the flesh.

God's promise to us is that if we allow Him to transform us, He will empower us to live supernaturally. The problem is that our core issues stand in the way of our moving into the supernatural. *Core beliefs* are the deeply rooted, oftentimes hidden foundational values that motivate our day-to-day lives. They create our perceptions of life. (Remember, our perceptions are how we see life or view the world.) So, in essence, they are what we filter all our information through. Our perceptions will either be clear and truthful or cloudy and contaminated by the influence of the substance of our hearts. Jesus said that what is within a man, in his heart, defiles him (Mark 7:20–23). I believe He was referring to our core values or beliefs. Restoration is only possible if we connect our core beliefs with our actions and allow God to change them by real encounters with His Spirit.

Are Your Beliefs True or False?

Our thoughts and experiences help us formulate our beliefs. They are formed as we choose direction for our life. God intervenes throughout our lives, often by sending people who represent Him to show us the way to go—but we have to choose which path to take. I cannot spend my life blaming my parents or anyone else because I don't like the path I am on. I must take responsibility for what I believe and allow God to bring change in my life.

Let's face it. Everything we experience as we grow up does not represent God's nature and His goodness. All of creation is twisted by sin, and sin stems from the choice we make to go our own way. If we choose our way over God's way, the truth is distorted, and we open the door for false beliefs to form in us. These beliefs rise out of our painful and disappointing experiences, especially when we get stuck in our emotional pain. In other words, this ungodly way of believing takes root in us because of the way we adapt to pain and suffering.

A *false belief* is the misrepresentation of God's truth. For instance, I can tell you "God loves you" all day long, but until you are able to absorb and experience His love firsthand, my words may be practically meaningless to you. If you are still stuck in your pain (which

could come from childhood or other experiences), then you will
define love on the basis of your pain. Your assumption may be that
no one could love you, not even God. Get it? If you have a hole in
your heart, you will not be able to contain the goodness of God, even
if He pours it in daily.

Our beliefs reflect what is in our heart. The Bible refers to the
heart over eight hundred times, describing it in many ways—from its
evilness to its existence as a vehicle for trusting God. Scripture points
to the heart as the center of the will, and since our will and motivations compel us to live, knowing whether our will is broken is key
in helping us discover our beliefs. If our heart/will is broken because
of emotional trauma, even in adulthood we may be prone to defend
the tenderness of our wound. Our defensive actions may include
promiscuity, drivenness, insecurity, anger, rejection, and a host of
other behaviors, all of which are a reflection of the hurt that has not
been overcome and the false beliefs that generate such conduct.

For instance, I was sexually abused by an older male teenager in
my neighborhood when I was ten years old. I knew instinctively the
incident was wrong and very shameful, but because my relationship
with my parents was unsafe, I did not feel I could share the situation
with them. I grew up believing that everything bad that happened
to me was my fault. I believed that I was a bad kid. So even when I
was accosted by someone during a vulnerable time like adolescence, I
internalized that I was deserving of the experience. The consequences
of this experience caused me to live with a broken heart for many
years. I carried this belief of worthlessness into my adulthood. It
controlled my perception of my identity until I was healed.

This type of experience conditions us to live with a broken heart
and prevents us from receiving from God. It plays a major role in
what we believe and our need for transformation. The fact that false
beliefs prevent supernatural transformation is the reason why this
chapter and the next are on discovering what we believe about God,
Satan, self, and others. Each section builds an understanding of
how these particular beliefs impact our ability to know and experience God and the people around us. The goal is to interact with the

subject so that you develop a personal and specific understanding of what you believe. Gaining insight about your personal beliefs is rewarding because as God transforms you, it brings freedom and empowerment to be the person He purposed you to be.

False Beliefs about God That Prevent Supernatural Transformation

God is a Father to those who know Him in His true nature. He is love, and He wants us to experience all the benefits of His love. But if we are not clear on the goodness of His nature, all of our beliefs will be tainted. It is like growing up in a home with a loving father who balances his embraces with firm discipline for our protection. That supportive environment empowers us to know we are secure and teaches us to mature. But the problem is that many of us did not grow up with a good foundation of a father's love in our homes. Therefore, our image of God as a good, loving Father who seeks to empower us to live a life full of blessings is distorted by an unhealthy relationship with our earthly father. This unfortunate reality lays a foundation for false beliefs that trickle down to every experience in our lives.

False Belief #1: God Is Responsible for Everything Bad in My Life

It is not uncommon for us to rationalize suffering by blaming someone else for the pain. Typically, we put more blame on the Creator than anyone else. The accusation is that He has irresponsibly handled the calamity of fallen man. We put Him on trial for everything wrong in our lives, yet we try to make it sound really nice when we speak these accusations. We utter things like "I just don't understand why God would allow this innocent person to suffer. Where is God in all this mess? Why doesn't God heal today?" Ultimately, we shift the issue to blaming God by labeling the struggle as mysterious and unapproachable. Our beliefs are stated so that we tiptoe around the feelings of those who are suffering. We don't want to offend. We refer to Job as the hallmark case study to defend our putting God on trial. If the hurt or suffering is deep, we are often bitter toward God.

I am offering insight into why we are separated from God in our affliction; I am not trying to explain why some tragedies defy our wisdom. I do not believe all suffering makes sense to us in the present age because we wrangle with the issues with an imperfect and self-centered viewpoint. Looking for the "why" to resolve the "what" often creates more anguish in the face of those who are searching for comfort. Nevertheless, we must choose either to get busy living or get busy dying.

Job's case reflects the spiritual war that takes place in preserving the souls of men. God wanted to sustain and uphold Job, and Satan battled to destroy him. Through it all, Job eventually discovered that God was good and dependable. We no longer live in the days of Job; we live in a new era of time. We have access to so much more than Job, yet we still put God on trial.

The Lord's nature is to restore, not destroy. Jesus became the Man with the plan to redeem us. God is into *real* solutions. Have you ever wondered why it took God four thousand years to unfold His plan of salvation? He was setting up a real solution that would restore our fallen condition. He was not interested in leaving us to resolve our pain and suffering on our own. He penetrated our world, planet earth, in the form of a real man who demonstrated healing, deliverance, and salvation for real suffering. The works of healing and deliverance were the key means by which He set up His kingdom on earth. I am not sure how that registers in your book, but I call healing and delivering the sick a good thing.

The misconception of many is that God is unjust. Some Christians as well as non-Christians blame Him for much of the suffering in the world today. For example, I have many people ask me why God allows sickness, pain, and suffering. The core of this question is filled with an accusation. All who deem God as unjust also believe He is responsible for evil. God did not create evil nor does He sponsor it.

Evil exists on this planet because we (human beings) collaborate with the devil, who is the ultimate perpetrator of all evil.

You may retort, "Why does God allow evil to remain?" The answer to that is, God has a plan, plan B, since man messed up His initial plan, plan A, by choosing to sin. What we want is to have all our responsibility eliminated in one snap of His fingers—*poof*, all evil is gone. But we have a role to play. After all, man invited evil into the world, so if God were to abolish all evil, He would have to take away our free will as well. But that won't happen. As long as there is evil in this world, our nature will be able to be corrupt because man has a will. God addressed the force of evil at Calvary. From the foundation of the world He planned for Jesus to be put on the cross, to dethrone the forces of evil and reverse the curse of darkness that corrupted us in the garden. (See Rev. 13:8.)

God does not allow evil to remain. He has equipped us new covenant believers with the force of light to expose it and remove it. That is our responsibility as agents of truth and light. I like how Luke recorded the prayer of Jesus for Peter's mother-in-law (Luke 4:39). Luke said that Jesus rebuked her fever. Why would He rebuke a fever? The reason is that it did not belong in creation or in her body (as a daughter of Abraham and child of God). How different would the world be if we took the same attitude of Christ and removed everything that did not belong in creation?

Yet we mumble and shrug our responsibility. Not only do we not want to take responsibility for ourselves, but in our generation, we have also become very impatient, demanding instant gratification. We think the world should revolve around us. So when things go wrong and we face suffering, we either look for reasons to alleviate the symptoms or we blame something or someone else for our problems. We go searching for pain relief. If we do not find it when we pray, then we say prayer does not work. Is it possible that something could be missing in our prayer? I find that God not only meets us with various levels of faith, but He always meets us if we persevere. Perseverance is a lost attribute in our quick-fix society. We want everything now.

Unlike the disciples spoken of in the Bible whose suffering came for righteousness sake, much of our suffering comes from disobedience and rebellion because of the lifestyles that we choose to live. We live as if there are no boundaries in life. We push ourselves, striving for success, and when we run into pain, we medicate it so that it does not surface. We have no peace because we do not rest. Eventually, our world comes crashing down around us, and we are confused as to why it happens.

So should God be held liable for our wrong choices? The simple answer is no. Yet God has always taken responsibility for our suffering by providing alternatives for our restoration. He entered into our sinful condition, seeking to redeem us from ourselves. He has not only taken responsibility for our sin, He desires to remove its consequences in our lives. He is providing a way for us to have abundant life, rescuing us from our mortal destruction. His plan of restoration is full scale, offering us power to overcome the destructive weight of our sin and the sins of others against us.

This plan includes an essential ingredient—our willingness. The Lord always allows us to choose our path. If we choose Him, we are promised abundant life, and if we rebel against Him, we must face a life full of destruction. I don't know about you, but I am learning to choose life!

God is not responsible for all the bad in my life. Regardless of how it got there—my sin, the sins of others, or the deceiver himself—I have to choose to deal with it. My Bible tells me that no matter what circumstances I face, the Lord has an answer and a plan to redeem me. My prayer is that all unbelief be replaced with the truth that God has a plan to redeem us. It can begin with you and me. So I ask you to join me in letting go of the accusations against Him and discovering how He wants to transform your misery into triumph.

False Belief #2: God Is Not Moving among His People Today

Some struggle to see the handiwork of God in the midst of His people. Those who acquiesce to this lie believe that God is not saving us. They are actually saying one of two things: (1) God is not able or willing to meet us, so His involvement is non-existent; or (2) He is not alive, perpetuating His plan on the earth, and thus He is dead. These people assume that God has more important things to think about, like issues of eternity. Assuming He is not concerned about us leads us to believe that He is distant and unapproachable. This perception is very dangerous because it portrays God as harsh and judgmental.

It is a direct lie that God has rejected us because He is mad at us. This is not His nature. God does not give up on us like we give up on ourselves or each other. The story would be over if God had given up on us. There would be no world because we would have destroyed ourselves. If we follow that line of thinking, He has wasted a lot of time and resources to prepare His people. Let me explain.

We would be foolish to think God set up this plan, the atonement of Jesus, so that He could use it as a license to torture us. No way; it is just the opposite. He set up this elaborate plan and prepared us for it so that we would win. Through His grace, we can face our struggles and have absolute victory, along with receiving the benefits of all His promises.

God is the initiator. He sees everything in terms of restoration. He did not wait for us to come to our senses; He was on the move, setting restoration in order after the fall of mankind. He pursues us and does not give up on us. God's movement is clearly visible throughout history. Every generation receives a visitation. It is evident to me that He is visiting us today. We have a responsibility to take action on His move in our lives. But self-pity can prevent us from moving forward and taking action as God moves, because our eyes are on our weaknesses.

This kind of mindset causes us to stand by and watch the works of God take place and feel that we cannot enter into them because we are not good enough. None of us qualify for this battle on our own; we are only able to take action as a result of His strength and character, not ours. I can only win my personal battles by leaning on Him and allowing Him to give me strength, which is true for everyone.

That is not to say that God does not have any expectations of us. His plan is simple. He gives life for life. His covenant with us is built upon His everlasting commitment to His people. He has given the life of His Son as the seal of His commitment to meet us in our suffering. Our responsibility is to yield the control of our lives to Him. This surrender is the *divine exchange*—He gave His life full of righteousness so that we can exchange with Him our life full of messes. In this way, He restores our life back to us.

The move of God starts when we realize our need for Him. That usually happens because He sends a messenger (another person) who wakes us up and brings us back to the truth so that real reconciliation can take place. The exchange process begins when we admit we made a royal mess of things. I will never forget sitting up in my bed, telling my wife the revelation the Lord gave me of how I opened the door for my physical sickness through my lifestyle of drivenness. I discovered rebellion and fear were driving me more than grace and faith. It was a very freeing revelation when I came to understand that my problems were not just some fluke thing that had befallen me. God placed messengers in my life that I could have easily ignored, but I knew that my life depended upon listening to them.

The message of restoration came to me from people. They gave me an explanation of how I "got broke" and how I could "get fixed." Their intervention was an act of grace that God used to reach into my situation and transform me. I could not change myself or heal myself, but I did have to cooperate with the process. Rather than discounting their message, I paid close attention, and I learned how to exercise my faith. The message was the same one Jesus preached—I had made a mess and He had a plan to clean it up. The move of God in our lives is sometimes so simple that we ignore it.

The one thing that I realized in the process was that God was not going to overhaul my life without my permission—I needed to take responsibility for the chaos I had created. I learned that we fall into passivity if we do not believe we have a responsibility in our restoration. When being passive, we form this belief: *There is no hope, so why try to overcome? God has forgotten me, and I am doomed to suffer and die.* Passivity is self-pity sucking us down the tube of despair. The voice of the enemy becomes powerful in this false belief because we are confused by Satan's accusation of God's unfaithfulness. The enemy screams in our ear, "God does not care about you; give up and die!" If we yield to this lie of passivity—that it is better to not try than to try and fail—then we play right into the hand of our enemy. He wants us to believe we have no power or right to walk in God's overcoming strength.

God demonstrated His will regarding our weak condition and our inability to restore ourselves by giving us Jesus Christ, His Son. This gift is His intervention for mankind. The conclusion of Jesus' gospel message of liberation was to leave His presence here on earth. No sooner did He leave than He gave us the Holy Spirit. The Holy Spirit now makes the continuation of the gospel possible and real for all who believe. He is alive and He is moving today. I see Him transform people all the time. It is funny to me as I look back, because before my own personal transformation, I rarely saw Him transform others. But since I've started believing the transforming process is real, I witness it on a regular basis.

False Belief #3: God Is Unpredictable in His Intervention with His People

This belief lends to the conclusion that God is haphazard. Some believers say things like, "God's ways are mysterious; who can know them?" or "God helps those who help themselves," or "God's ways do not make sense." Out of this mentality grow things like random acts of kindness or justified anger toward God.

People clinging to this lie are confused about the authority extended to them in Christ. They refuse to believe that God is inviting them to be a vessel of His awesome power and strength.

If God's acts are random, then He is double-minded about His plan to redeem us. Of course, that is not so. Since the beginning of time, He has instilled a plan to provide for and perpetuate His goodness. The problem is not a lack of clarity regarding God's intervention, but a deficiency on the part of man to appropriate the goodness of God. I know from personal experience, while we are busy blaming Him, we are missing out on the fulfillment of His promises. In my case, the angrier I became about my pitfall, the further I separated myself from the goodness of God. Using rational, current-day, "right" theology, I blamed my suffering on the fall of man.

This is the same argument that the man lying by the pool of Bethesda used during his interview with Jesus. When the crippled man said, "'I have no man to help me into the pool to get healed when the water is stirred,'" in essence he was saying, "Life is not fair because other people get blessed and God passes me over" (John 5:7). I find the Lord's response amazing: Jesus bypasses the man's pity party and asks him if he wants to be healed. This question appears cruel, but through it, Jesus makes a powerful point about God's restoration. It is available for all; the only requirement is to say yes.

Believing that God's actions are haphazard produces pain management therapy: we cannot predict whether God is going to be angry, so we take some painkillers and walk with a hobble. But Jesus did not address the sick and dying people of His day in this manner. He reached into their death-filled mentalities and extended life to them. Life is what I needed in my situation when I was sick and dying. I did not need someone to sit by me and stroke my head. I needed God to reach into my situation and restore me. If all I had done was seek to manage my pain, I would have been left to my own power and ability. I needed the supernatural moving of the Holy Spirit to intervene in my situation. I needed God's touch in this life, not the next one in eternity.

Furthermore, we resist the move of God by reducing the atonement to eternal security. We relegate the provision of the living God to a mere passageway into another life. The gospel of Jesus Christ becomes powerless because we take no risk to believe it and apply it to our everyday problems. If others do happen to believe the message of His healing, delivering power, we label them a peripheral group of extremist Christians, and we pronounce, "That's not real!"

I hear people say that those people who believe in the power of the Holy Spirit for today are caught up in a movement. I say yes they are; it's called the movement of the Holy Spirit. It is the same movement that started the church and it continues to this day. If God used miracles, signs, and wonders to start the church, wouldn't you agree that it is logical for Him to use the same thing to continue the church? The method that worked for Jesus should be our focus too. Either Jesus was the Son of God and reflected the will of the Father, or Jesus was messing up God's plan to teach us hard lessons through our sickness and suffering.

Favoritism is another element to this ungodly belief. The thought is that only a certain group of people get to experience the blessings of God, that God's plan involves an elite people. Therefore, the secular world views the Christian God as exclusive. But although His Word clearly states that His plan was to prepare chosen people to bring the gospel to the world, our heavenly Father is not interested in giving the advantage to one group over another, nor does He value one of His children over another. If He restored other generations, He will do the same thing in this generation. His Word says that He is the same, yesterday, today, and forever (Heb. 13:8). God desires that none perish. If certain individuals or groups feel they are excluded, it is because they choose to hang onto their discrimination built on a victimized mentality. The Bible says that we cannot serve two masters (Matt. 6:24). It's either the Savior of the world or the prince of darkness—we can take our pick. But, as the old saying goes, "You can't have your cake and eat it too."

The bottom line is if we are not experiencing the life-saving, awesome, overwhelming, real power of God, then it is because we believe but are unwilling to move with Him. The lack of His presence in our lives or the authority to solve the world's problems is not His fault. It is ours, because of our choices. His authority in our lives is diminished because we subject ourselves to a lifestyle of compromise, driven by our need to be in control. I know that as long as I run my life my way, the end result will be destruction. I found out that I cannot live life without abiding in His presence daily. My experience along the way has been that God does prove His Word to me but I choose to doubt its validity. There were people with the power of the Holy Spirit working all around me when I crashed. I had too much pride to admit I was needy—I could not allow that side of me to show. That was the problem.

God is often speaking, but we have plugged our ears with self-pity or disappointment so that we do not recognize His voice. God is not moved by our disappointment or self-pity. For example, our kids do the same thing to us. They come to us whining about their boo-boos but then refuse the medicine that will bring healing because it hurts when applied. We do the same thing with God. He says repent, but we say no because that hurts. Our cry is, "Give me pity, not discipline."

God is not random; He is deliberate in His redemption with us. He made His plan of salvation a public event for the whole world to see and experience. He does not hide His goodness *from* us; He hides it *for* us. We are called to discover the greatness of God as we seek after Him. He is so active, preparing, establishing, and reaping His Word in the earth today. Those who experience this reality are those who yield to Him.

I offer this strong voice of correction because I watch people who are suffering go round and round with God over their misery—and I know what that agony feels like. Remember, I am writing this as a survivor and overcomer of self-inflicted infirmity, not as an observer. I have been there; I know what it is like to question God and wrestle with the issue of evil in the world. God's plan to restore you may seem confusing, but know this: God is not at fault, and the quicker you stop putting Him on trial, take Him off the witness stand, and come before Him in submission, the quicker you will find rest in His presence. The Lord is your only hope! All others are just vehicles of creation that point to Him, your Creator. I encourage you to learn to trust Him rather than fight Him.

False Beliefs about Satan That Prevent Supernatural Transformation

Our false beliefs about God distort our understanding of how the enemy, Satan, works in our lives. Many blame God for the things

Satan does. Some blame Satan for things they are responsible for doing. This cycle spirals on and on until we take an active role in discerning the truth about our enemy. I don't intend to focus on him, but he must be identified and removed if we plan to live victoriously in Christ.

False Belief #1: Satan Is a Myth

Recently my wife and I sat in astonishment as we watched a woman on TV talk about her new book. She was being interviewed by one of the major network morning shows. No, her book was not about the newest cookbook or parenting modality. It was about the activity of the occult. In casual clothing and with a grandmotherly twist, she revealed how the occult was no longer an issue depicted by movies like *The Wizard of Oz*. The occult is common and accepted in our society; it is the presence of darkness masqueraded as light. The sad thing about the program we watched was that many Christians and countless others who saw it have little discernment about the seriousness of what her book and life represent to the Christian church.

We think of Satan as a toothy red imp who walks around in a 36-inch costume on October 31 in celebration of Halloween. Many theologians and everyday churchgoers alike have reduced him to a mythical figure of ancient times. Those who suppose the devil to be a real figure, influencing their lives with oppression and sickness, hold no credibility and are considered antiquated and borderline crazy.

What did Jesus believe about His adversary, the devil? The key question is, did Jesus believe in the existence of a personal devil and his demons, or was His conception only of impersonal but powerful forces of evil in the universe? The way we answer this question will determine our true belief about the devil and the spiritual world. If we believe that the encounter of Christ with the devil was mythical, then we will see the devil and his presence in this real world as mythical. However, if we believe the Matthew 4 account that the Holy Spirit led Jesus into the wilderness, into a face-to-face confrontation with the devil (vv. 1–10), then we will determine that the prince of the air truly has an impact in this present world.

Explaining Christ and Satan's direct confrontation as a myth reduces Jesus' ministry and miracles to the same. Yet we know from the Bible that Christ spent a great amount of time casting out demons and teaching His disciples about the reality of the spirit world. He did not shy away from exposing the works of Satan or even from taking his own followers head on when necessary.

From the time of His conception until He hung on the cross before the world, the devil's goal was to destroy the Son of God. The last words of Christ to His disciples included instructions to cast out devils (Mark 16:17). On numerous occasions, Jesus brought deliverance from evil spirits and healing to the body in the same breath. There's no doubt that Jesus believed the enemy was real.

Remember, I am not trying to glamorize the devil. I think His accomplishments are very overrated. He is often given credit he does not deserve. But I believe that if we act as if he does not exist, we may fall prey to him unknowingly. The apostle Paul knew we needed to on guard against Satan; he said to Timothy, his son in the faith, that we can be taken captive by the enemy if we are not careful (2 Tim. 2:26).

Even C.S. Lewis, one of the most notable scholars of our time, wrote in his book *The Screwtape Letters* that one of the greatest tricks of Satan is to deceive us into believing that the devil and demons do not exist.[1] I can only add that if Jesus agrees the devil is a very real opponent, then we need to learn to war against him as Jesus did. (We'll be learning about spiritual warfare in a later chapter.)

False Belief #2: I Am Saved; I Have No Evil in My Life

The story I am about to tell you is absolutely real. If I do not tell it, then some will quickly write off my admonishment regarding the works of the devil in the lives of believers as being the extreme rare occasion rather than more frequent. My wife and I were attending church one Sunday morning in a small, quiet town about an hour and half south of Atlanta, Georgia. We drove by some friends' house on the way to church and to our surprise there was police tape surrounding their property. We wrote it off as a possible break-in and robbery. That scenario alone would be devastating enough, considering the potential damage; but it would be an afternoon in the park compared to the reality that had taken place in the middle of the night in the home of these born-again, church-going, children's ministry volunteers, and proud parents of two sweet little children. This thirty-something couple had recently remodeled their home, and these two energetic owners had performed all the work themselves—but that night a murder had transpired there.

The intruder was not a rogue criminal searching for unsuspecting prey; he was the husband of the lovely wife who was choked to death. She was destroyed at the hands of her childhood lover because of an argument that had spun out of control. The gore does not stop there. After he choked her, he then proceeded to develop a plan for the demise of the entire family. He ran downstairs and turned on the gas oven, supposing to destroy the children too; then he ran upstairs to turn a gun on himself. Later, his children found him and fled to safety, making a collect call to a relative for help.

Yes, this happened, and yes, it is real. It reflects how even well-intentioned, dedicated Christians can struggle with evil, whether to this degree or a lesser one.

This information is crucial to understanding how to win the race. Satan prowls about looking for weakness in the lives of believers. He very subtly brings his influence into our minds by planting seeds of doubt and confusion within our belief system. As we encounter painful or traumatic situations while we are growing up, the enemy seeks to take up residence in our pain. He does this by shaping what we believe about our suffering. His technique for imparting darkness into our souls is to leave deposits of fear, envy, anger, bitterness, rejection, and shame after the hurtful or distressing event. What happens over time is that wrong values get mixed in with right values—creating a cohabitation of good and evil on the inside of a person.

Let me help you get a visual picture of how good and evil cohabit. Imagine a person—body, soul, and spirit—as though he were a house that is very much lived in. He has "stuff" everywhere, displayed on shelves, in cabinets, on every surface, and in every other available nook and cranny. Some of these things were purchased, some were received as hand-me-downs from relatives, and some came from who knows where (they are junk and should be thrown away). However, for various reasons, the owner cannot seem to part with any of them. Eventually, the person decides to redecorate the house and needs to part with some of the stuff in order to complete the renovation. But what does he do? He just sticks that old stuff somewhere out of sight—under beds, in closets, in the garage, and in the attic. And so, although he has not actually removed the old junk, the appearance of the house has changed.

This scenario is similar to what happens inside some of us as believers. We decide to follow God, which for most people means becoming a Christian and joining a church. However, for many of us, our decision to follow Christ is like our decision to redecorate our house. We purchase a Bible and start going to church, and we might start talking, behaving, and dressing differently. But what happens to our old beliefs after we've repented at the altar? Where do the beliefs go? Do they just pass away when we invite Jesus into our hearts? Well, maybe that happens for some of us. But, as for the rest of us, we shove those beliefs into the attic or to the back of our closet, scoot them over on the shelves, or build a new storeroom for them out back. Granted, there might be a few of us who are smart: we hold a yard sale to get rid of our unwanted junk or we give it to charity. However, unless we start completely from scratch, we will always have old stuff that remains.

The next step is to put up new wallpaper, a fresh coat of paint, a new floor covering, and maybe add some landscaping on the outside of our house to help it "appear" new. (I'm still talking about our body and soul.) Do you get the picture of your own "house" now?

Although we may be Christians, this is how we may also house evil. Those of us who are in this situation feel that there is a constant battle taking place on the inside, and we may be tormented by it. So we keep ourselves busy or self-medicated to block out the torment. The means by which we self-medicate may be socially acceptable; for example, we could use eating, shopping, or working as a coping mechanism. On the other hand, we might commit shameful acts such as drinking excessive amounts of alcohol, abusing prescription medications, using illegal drugs, or viewing pornography. Meanwhile, as we live in denial, the enemy is taking up residence in our soul— our mind (our thoughts), will, and emotions—and he is gaining a stronghold. The old beliefs are still in place. We just covered them up with religious activity.

The enemy's presence can grow to the level of gaining a monopoly in our thinking, influencing our every decision. For instance, do you do the things you know that you shouldn't do way too often, even to the extent that you feel out of control of your own body? Do you find that no sooner have you made your declaration of freedom than you are once again yielding to the kingdom of darkness? This is a good sign your enemy has gained a stronghold in your life. He has fortified his presence in your life, with your cooperation, so much so that now you are starting to believe that this is who you really are. You are characterized as depressed, angry, nervous, rejected, and envious—all of which came as you collaborated with evil.

This is why the apostle Paul spent so much time instructing the young churches he ministered to about the devices of the enemy. He warned the church of Ephesus to be aware of the spiritual war that is taking place in the heavenly realms. Paul was so keenly aware of this war that his message to us was, if we are not careful, we will fight with each other rather than the real enemy. (See Eph. 6:12.) The early church was intensely aware of the spiritual battle at hand. They put their lives on the line, knowing that at any point the enemy's persecution could cost them their security in Christ. Early followers of Christ gathered in the homes of fellow believers to strengthen the brethren in the battle against the enemy. Guess who won? The apostle John records in Revelation 12:11 that the believers overcame Satan by the blood of the lamb and the word of their testimony, and they loved not their lives unto death.

Let me illustrate the truth about our enemy. Recently my wife summoned me outside to the back of our home on a Saturday morning. I was tired and groggy from recent travels, so I made my way outside with very little pep in my step. But when she alerted me that there was a copperhead snake under our deck, the same place our children had been playing the weekend before, all of a sudden my adrenaline kicked in, and I was on full alert.

There the enemy was, slithering around in my territory.

Now, I am not a snake lover, and I especially don't like the ones that can kill my children. Being an outdoors kind of guy, I quickly set in motion my strategy—kill, and do it quickly.

Planning to hold the snake down and behead him, I fetched a long rake and an axe. I then executed my plan with swiftness. In no time at all, there the beast lay, severed from the neck up. I picked up the long body and carried it away to be discarded.

When I came back to get the head, to my amazement, the snake still had the audacity to think he could bite me and poison me. I was dumbfounded that this beheaded reptile had any life left within him.

This scenario exemplifies the truth about our enemy, Satan. Even though Jesus beheaded and dethroned Satan, he still possesses the power to deceive us, should we choose to let him. If we submit to his enticing ways, he can get into our heads, as he did with Eve in the garden. (See Gen. 3:1–6.) If we get too close, he can bite us. He can even kill us if we allow his poison (wrong beliefs and thoughts) to remain.

The good news is that the enemy is beheaded. We need to realize that Jesus overcame him and set us up to do the same through the Word, Jesus' name, and His blood. We have authority over Satan because Jesus endowed us with victory. We no longer have to be afraid of the devil. If we let him in or open a door unknowingly, we simply need to repent and run to the Lord for help. He will give us victory over our enemy every time.

Prayer:

Father, I ask you to reveal to me any false beliefs in my life. Show me the beliefs I hold to be true that prevent me from moving forward with You. Give me clarity about any thought patterns that are fueling my actions and preventing me from receiving Your Word. Make Your beliefs real to me. Guide me through this exchange process. Expose all lies in my life. Replace these lies with the truth of Your Word and, according to Your revealed truth, change my thinking, speaking, and acting. Give me strength to lay down everything that I am holding onto that prevents me from receiving this message. I want to live according to Your precious promises. Fill me with Your Spirit so that I can move through this process with discernment. I pray in the name of Jesus Christ, my Lord. Amen.

CHAPTER 4

YOU ARE WHAT YOU BELIEVE, PART 2

Getting Real about the Truth

IF GOD IS OUT OF ORDER AND WE ARE BLIND TO THE oppression of the devil, then our perception about who we are will be very warped. In a forest, a tree that cannot receive sunlight will naturally bend as it seeks light and, over time, will grow crooked. We do the same thing when our beliefs about God are twisted: we seek light and fulfillment apart from Him and, as a result, our identity as a person is twisted. I don't want that to be your life story, so we're going to continue looking at more misconceptions that prevent supernatural transformation, starting with people's false beliefs about self.

False Belief #1: My Sin, My Sin—It's Only My Sin

The issue of sin is inaccurately portrayed when churches limit it to blatant, inappropriate acts or behaviors such as lying, adultery, stealing, or murder (the ones listed in the Ten Commandments)

or when churches simplify its definition to be "an inappropriate
response to a valid need." While sin does include the wrong behaviors and while the preceding definition sounds nice and is palatable
and even partly accurate, both of these depictions fall short of biblical
truth. Jesus did not mince words when it came to defining the issues
surrounding the fallen nature of man. He included in His definition
of sin the connection to the evil one, Satan. When confronting the
Jews for their erroneous beliefs, Christ reminded them that they were
of their father, the devil (John 8:44). In essence, He was saying that
their religious pride was enhanced by a spiritual stronghold which
was developed by the presence of the devil in their thinking. In other
words, they were living according to lies.

How is it possible to seem so righteous outwardly and at the same
time to be so far from God deep within? Because "the lie" we fell
for in the beginning says we don't need a god, let alone the God,
our Creator. So in this sense, the religious elite are like many of us:
we both seek to live as if there is no need for God. And to live a life
independent from God is nothing less than to live a life of sin.

Sin includes a much broader range of beliefs and behaviors than
just those that don't exemplify a need for Christ. So, although this list
of traits is not all-inclusive, we must recognize the following attributes
in our definition of sin: fear, independence, bitterness, unforgive-
ness, envy, jealousy, self-hatred, rejection, anger, religious pride,
and shame. Oftentimes we call characteristics like these "emotional
problems." We do not recognize them as sin. Why? Because, many
believers in the body of Christ would think we were condemning
them if we said that a quality such as *fear* is "sin." Yet the Word of
God plainly says that whatever is not of faith is sin (Rom. 14:23).
The validity of this scripture is without question, for any behavior
that leads to torment *must* stem from sin. Perhaps another way to put
it is to say that anything that doesn't produce dependence on God
produces separation from Him.

God's Word encourages you to view yourself as righteous, clean,
and acceptable because of the provision of Christ. Any thought or
action that causes you to doubt that reality is sin. It is sin to disagree

with the Word of God about what it says about you. Even if you have been shamed as a child by physical abuse or you now live in an abusive marriage, it is a contradiction for you to hold a shameful perception of yourself if God's Word declares otherwise.

We become separated from God when we agree with sin and the kingdom of darkness. It is like the trickle-down effect that occurs in caves as water drips down the walls, forming rock sculptures. The flow of the water shapes the rock, which becomes hard. In the same way, the more we consent to the power of sin, the more it will shape our lives and cause our hearts to become hard toward God. Paul admonishes us in his letter to the Hebrews to throw off any sin "which so easily besets us" (Heb. 12:1). It is natural to sin; likewise, it is supernatural to walk in dependence upon God.

Let me cut to the chase. I believe that the force of sin is linked to a spiritual force backed up by the kingdom of darkness. Fear is both an emotion and a spirit, a demonic force. If I agree with fear, then I set in motion a process of learning in my soul that causes me to agree with that negative emotion and open the door to the presence of the spirit of fear in my life. That process can produce in me deep oppression over the course of time. Eventually, it may show up in my body in the form of pain to the stomach or other internal area like the heart. This is a reality for many born-again believers.

If we walk in sin, then we walk under the influence of the kingdom of darkness. If we walk in obedience to God's Word, then we walk under the influence of the kingdom of light. God has given us mercy in the gift of Christ to empower us to walk in the light. I write this to encourage you, not to scare you. I realize that just because we practice walking in the light one day, we do not undo the course of disobedience in our life that has formed over many years. It takes a process of application and appropriation to turn around the force of darkness and remove the consequences of sin. However, as we practice walking in the light each day, over the course of time we will be changed.

Many people accept the lie that the force of sin at work within them is who they are. They actually identify themselves with sinful characteristics of the kingdom of darkness. The lies that we have accepted from the enemy are so casual and readily acceptable that they often go unnoticed. For example, in describing ourselves, we say, "I am just high-strung" or "I am a little crabby; so what?" or "It's not a big deal if I am easily upset" or "Defensiveness is my defense mechanism" or "Everybody's got an addiction or two," all of which soften the idea of how darkness is ruling our lives.

Our only hope when it comes to sin and overthrowing the kingdom of darkness that seeks to control our lives is the application of the gospel of Jesus Christ. His life, death, and resurrection serve as our vicarious way of exchanging a life of sin, death, and despair. He gives me hope because He faced and overcame everything I face. I have it if I am willing to receive it. Bless God, that is a remarkable trade! He carries the weight of my sin and I, in turn, receive His righteousness. I am required to yield to Him and allow Him to remove all darkness.

For me, I discovered that I do not have the ability to examine my own heart and make corrections. I learned in this process that being open to others around me to speak into my life is critical. Allowing people that I trust to walk me gently through my struggles is a great asset. No man is an island. If you want to know how you show up in life, then you need to be bold and ask your family. They will tell you truthfully, and what you do with their insight is between you and God.

Sin does not just go away. It must be removed and cleansed. Just because I came to Christ thirty years ago at summer camp does not mean I am living in the righteousness of my Lord. The Bible tells me that I am the righteousness of God through faith in Christ Jesus (Rom. 3:22), but my actions may not be exemplifying that righteousness. Walking in righteousness is an active process. The Holy Spirit brings conviction and I yield to Him. The Lord cleanses me and renews my mind, replacing the old man with a new one who desires the heart of God.

The closer we get to the Lord, the more refinement is required. It is like viewing a painting from a distance. You cannot see the brush strokes until you get close. God continues to transform us because it is to our benefit. Our learning to obey Him is something that excites Him. He even stands to attention when we obey. Remember, Jesus stood as Stephen was martyred (Acts 7:55–56), not because it was a thrilling experience but to honor the obedience of a triumphant saint.

False Belief #2: I Am Unworthy of God's Provision

I caught a recent blurb from a national news service that said Americans will spend $750 million on self-help books this year (the year I am writing this book) and more than $1 billion on motivational speakers. Not only will Americans turn to these venues for answers, but they will also take college classes. In fact, more than 100 colleges now offer classes in positive psychology—the science of happiness. A psychologist reported that with so many resources focused on achieving happiness, we should all be brimming with joy.

I find the opposite in the lives of a large number of churchgoers who are struggling. I find deep despair rather than happiness or a confidence of restoration. Their hopelessness is built on their conclusion that because they failed to live a victorious life, they disqualified themselves from the blessings of God. I have found myself there on more than one occasion. Overcoming sin is an uphill climb on a slippery slope that seems impossible. Human potential in the fight against sin is like trying to fight a forest fire with a shovel. No sooner do you put out one fire than another one starts right behind it.

Although our inherent problem is our corrupt nature, I think the overall issue comes down to what we believe about the finished work of Christ on our behalf. It seems that for some, His offering is no more than fire insurance to escape the eternal flames of hell. But in order for the gospel message of our Messiah to become real to us, it must be more than a well-defined belief about eternity. So, I suggest we revisit the salvation message that we believed in the beginning.

Paul makes it clear that when we come to Christ we become new. He says that if we are in Christ, we are new creatures: "old things have passed away . . . all things have become new" (2 Cor. 5:17). What an awesome gift that is to be a new person! But there is unfinished business down in the depths of our souls. The goal is to move forward.

The key words in this scripture are *passed* and *become*; both words pertain to sanctification. What change did this conversion produce? Some say, because we are saved, everything works out without challenges; in other words, life is easy. Others say we have salvation, but that only applies to eternity. Their message is that life is a grind. Both points are incomplete and leave many asking, "Is this all there is?" Many never seek to progress beyond the salvation plan. There is more to the meaning of the scriptural principle of sanctification made by the apostle Paul.

Have you ever played sports or been involved in a challenging project, and no matter how hard you tried, deep in your heart you knew you would not win? I can still remember the thoughts of defeat I experienced as a football player when I looked at the scoreboard and knew that there was no way we could win the game. If you have experienced this type of "desperate perception," you know that it sets in motion a reaction. If we know we are going to lose, we give up before the game is even over.

The deep-gut feeling that "I am going to lose no matter how hard I try" is similar to the principle Paul is teaching about in the above scripture. If you know you are going to lose, you give up, but if you know you are going to win, you play with confidence. Paul is saying that once we become born again, we are transformed to win in life. We should no longer be controlled by the overwhelming feeling of loss. We win. And if we win, we should play the game differently— play to win. If we are new, made acceptable in God's eyes, then we should hold our heads up high and face the struggles in our lives, knowing that we are triumphant no matter what we face.

Sanctification is the key to freedom in Christ. It is the process of purging the soul from sin and renewing the mind through Christ. This principle is about transformation from the inside out. Granted, when I look in the mirror too long and stare at my flaws, all I see is flesh. But when I gaze into the loving eyes of my heavenly Father, I am reminded that I am a son of the Most High. Overcoming that deep-seated false belief that I am unworthy is not about an over-examination of my fleshly existence or turning my external behavior into self-righteous rigidity. It is about receiving a new nature from the supernatural Lord who lived a flawless life on a level that was above the will of the flesh. As I partake of His divine nature, He transforms my old nature, and I rise above the lowly, false belief that I do not deserve anything unless I crawl across beds of glass to get it.

If we are led to believe that acceptance comes from our appearance (how we dress and how we wear our hair) or by abstaining from vain and worldly things such as wearing make-up or jewelry, watching television or movies, or dancing, we will be in bondage to our legalism. These are all outward works that do not aid in the cleansing of our soul. They only mask what is really there. Most importantly, all removal of sin is an act of the Holy Spirit that is incorporated into our lives by faith. No one can remove sin without the work of the Holy Spirit.

The other extreme is that we offer followers a license to do whatever makes us happy because of grace. The mentality is *I do what makes me feel good about myself.* Paul addressed this issue in his letter to the Romans. He clearly says that to live as if there is no law would be a travesty. Grace does not provide a legal right to do whatever we want. We are provided grace as an act to empower us to become free from sin and its bondage. Grace is the power of God to transform an old, corrupt nature into a new, glorious nature. Why hang out at the trash dump if you are given a royal palace? Our sense of self-worth is not going to be raised by living in the shadows of the slums. We are worthy of this new citizenship for one reason and one reason alone. God rewarded us because of another Man's righteousness. I am somebody because the shed blood of Jesus Christ has cleansed me from sin. Behaving as if that never occurred dishonors His gift and discredits my new nature.

We are worthy by faith. Our faith is in the Lord, who conquered this worthlessness that stained us until now. I no longer base my right to the benefits of God on my goodness. I stand with boldness in His presence as a worthy son because the Son paid the price for me to be there. Whether you are bruised by legalistic attempts at conformity or you live by the fluffy leisure of lasciviousness, you are called to rise

to the occasion and accept Jesus for who He is—the Messiah who
took upon Himself the sin of the world. Find worthiness in Him. Let
Him convince you of your value, a value that is not founded on your
efforts but is rooted in the finished work of the One who lives in you.
If the devil can convince you of unworthiness, how much more can
the Savior of the world qualify you for worthiness?

False Belief #3: I Must Fix Myself and Be in Control

When unworthiness floods a person's life, his insecurities can drive
him to the point that he is constantly searching for safe harbor. I lived
that way for many years. In fact, I thought I had to drive myself so
that good things would come my way. I believed that I was responsible for making the "good life" happen and that, consequently, I had
to chase after my dreams. This limited view made life very difficult.
When problems arose, I believed I had to solve them. I thought I had
to control life and the endless influx of out-of-control circumstances
that pressed me every day. I was my own protector. My heavenly
Father became my assistant, not my God. The subconscious thought
was that He was following me where I wanted to go. I sought God
to get Him to do things for me and help me stay in control, and I
surmised that life was good. But the truth was, the end of this trail
yielded exhaustion and confusion. I learned that I am not God, nor
am I a god. I was created to be a follower of God.

This me-centered worldview creates a foundation of insecurity.
What happens when we get hit by a tidal wave? I find it difficult to
comprehend the force generated by the waves that the 2005 Southeast
Asia tsunami produced during the natural disaster that took place
there. The waves came ashore without any warning. It was a sunny
day at the beach. People were on vacation, children were playing,
and it was another carefree day. Then, out of nowhere destruction
struck. Suddenly, before anyone realized what was happening, the
waves came with such might that every life force in their path was
destroyed by the velocity and power of the moving water. People
everywhere panicked for their lives. It appeared as if they could not
find any place of safety. In the end, nothing in the water's path of

destruction lay untouched. For me, watching the fateful event on television was all too surreal.

How do we handle the forces of disaster that sweep through our lives? I panicked and ran for shelter. That is what most of us do. The truth is, we have no control over some of the things that come against us, nor do we have the capacity to handle everything that comes our way. But God does, and He always has a plan to use the most devastating things to our benefit if we allow Him to transform us in the process.

My way of fixing things is to remove whatever is in the way of my goals. If it is pain, I want relief; if it is marriage problems, I want a new mate; if it is my job, I want a new boss; if it is God, I want a new god. I cannot stand facing the mess I have created or the ones that others have created that I have become entangled in. I want a problem-free life, and when difficulties arise, I want to solve them my own way. But trying to fix situations myself only makes bad things worse. I cannot fix me or others. Trying to handle my problems in this manner is an illusion, something that appears real but is not.

Only God fixes people. All I can do is receive His help or assist others in doing the same thing. I cannot heal other people, but I can be a vessel of healing. The branch does not produce the tree; the tree produces the branch. Problems are fixed by facing them with grace. Walking in grace means allowing God to impart to us what we need to overcome everything we face. The most desperate situations have God's attention. The goal is to receive His goodness and then allow Him to use our difficulties to His advantage. God is faithful to finish what He starts. He walks us through the process, sometimes with instant change and sometimes by connecting each instance to one more step of victory. Remember, He is God and He is good. I find that His fixes last where mine come apart like plumbing held together with duct tape.

Recognizing that I cannot fix myself is a huge relief. Otherwise, I keep looking for the "right" fix. Fixing ourselves is our religion. Whom do we really trust? Our actions point to taking care of "me." However, the power of this realization is meaningless until we come to a place of deep surrender to God. I must realize I cannot control my life, nor will I ever be able to. The phrase "get control of my life" is a myth. My fleeting efforts to keep up with the unending pressures of life are like watching the famous comedienne Lucille Ball trying to work on a pie-making assembly line. The problems never quit coming, and my hands cannot move fast enough. It makes more sense to turn my life over to the engineer of the whole drama and plead His intervention on my behalf. If I am able to make any progress in the course of managing life, then it will flow out of my surrender to the Almighty, who offers me protection in His shadow and guidance on His path.

False Belief #4: To Receive, I Must Achieve

I made another discovery about myself. I realized I was trying to achieve in order to receive. This mistake stemmed from my false belief that my works move God to bless me. I did not realize I was loved and accepted because it was God's nature. His love and favor are gifts which cannot be earned. The goodness of God was made available to me as a birthright, not as a right of passage based upon performance. For example, in Genesis 32:24, 25, and 30, we see the patriarch Jacob wrestling with God in order to receive the blessing. However, according to Genesis 28:12–16, Jacob already had the blessing. So why was he wrestling? He believed he needed to prove his worthiness in order to receive the blessing, so he tried to manipulate God in exchange for it. In the end, God gave Jacob the blessing, but it came with a price—Jacob's hip was thrown out of joint (Gen. 32:25).

Our blessings have been paid for by the sacrificial life of Christ. It is not necessary to wrestle with God to receive them. I do not have to prove myself worthy of something that is freely offered to me by grace. I move into my authority by grace, learning to receive and apply the favor of God to my life. As a member of the supernatural race in the family of God, I am a son. It is my decision how I respond to my Father's leadership. I can either be a vessel of honor or dishonor.

Becoming a vessel of honor happens as a result of learning how to follow God. We bring honor to the Father because our actions lead to total dependence upon the Lord. Can you imagine what Abraham thought when the Lord told him to sacrifice his son Isaac? (See Gen. 22:2.) Offering up Isaac did not make good common sense, especially after all the time and labor spent in getting the boy. But scripture records Abraham did not hesitate; he obeyed. The end result was the most valuable lesson of Abraham's entire life—God is trustworthy (vv. 10–13). Our decisions should incorporate the same process: obey God at all costs and leave the results to Him. We are not required to become great men or women, but we are invited to become vessels of greatness. Our significance in this life comes from being a reflection of God's greatness as we yield ourselves to Him.

It is a privilege to be tried by the forces of evil and remain standing as a vessel of light. Even though darkness may cover us at times, we can endure running the course with our God. In fact, the most important aspect of the race is endurance. As John pointed out in his revelation to the seven churches in the first century, enduring to the end is the common thread of all faithful followers of our Lord (Rev. 2, 3); and it is he who endures to the end—not he who stands above the others—who shall be rewarded (Matt. 10:22). The goal is for all of us to cross the finish line together.

I remember an email someone sent me that was very inspirational. It was a Special Olympics event, and the setting was the 40-yard dash. The participants were a group of children who were physically challenged but spiritually shining. The race started, and they ran with all their might toward the finish line. The runners reached midpoint at varying levels when suddenly one child fell down, and down hard. As she lay there sobbing, the other runners, instead of carrying on without regard to their fallen foe, stopped and came to her aid. They consoled her and helped her to her feet. Then all at once without hesitation the group of youngsters locked arms at the elbow and made a chain. They walked forward and then began to trot in a single line until they finished the race, simultaneously crossing the finish line. Again I say, the goal in life is not to rise above others but to cross the finish line together to God's glory.

The most powerful force of transformation in the universe is the love of God. He demonstrated that love to us by giving us Christ. That love, the core of God's nature, is received because we see our need for it. He demonstrates His love to us in our weakness, not our self-sufficiency. If we are not careful, we can miss His love because we are too dependent on our perfectionist lifestyles. The apostle Paul said it this way, "I will rather glory in my weaknesses, that the power of Christ may overshadow me" (2 Cor.12:9). I concur. I say, "Bring on the love, Father God."

False Belief #4: I Cannot Change and Neither Does God Require Me to Change

Sometimes we do not see evidence of God's presence in our lives because we refuse to change. We find a seat on the back row at church and sit there hiding, hoping no one notices us. We drop out of the race altogether, believing that God does not require us to grow or change. But isn't it funny that Jesus Himself said to the religious folks of His day, "Either change or be thrown in the fire" (Matt. 23:13–33). We cannot flow in our divine purpose or experience the supernatural workings of God if we are not willing to change. In this sense, our lives are like a rubber hose. The more God desires to pour through us, the more we will be required to stretch. This stretching, or change, is good for us.

One thing that may prevent us from changing is shame. Why? Because shame creates separation between us and God. For example, when you feel shame, although you may desperately try to overcome the pull of the evil from within and live from God, you may continue to experience defeat if your core belief is that you should be ashamed of yourself. The gap between you and God will only grow wider. You may even begin to feel as though He has abandoned you. Being around fellow believers may then become difficult because you are living under such self-condemnation over this tormenting evil inside you that you begin to fear that if others discovered who you really are, they would reject you.

The condemnation that stems from shame causes many people to hide behind Christian masks. It is a real problem in the church. We have debilitating problems that we hide from others because of the image that goes along with the struggle. For instance, there are countless people who live in shame because they are on medications for anxiety, panic, phobias, or compulsive behavior. They want to be free, they think they should be free, but they have lost sight of how to be free. Please understand, I extend no condemnation to those who suffer in silence. Remember, my wife, who was married to the great Christian counselor/minister, was on antidepressants. However, at some point someone has to rock the boat that is going in a circle of despair.

Shame is like an infection on the skin. It is obvious. It festers and is unattractive. I can cover it and try to hide it, but that will not bring healing. We do the same thing with our shameful, sinful struggles in life. We find fig leaves to cover our problems, or we seek rational justifications to minimize the infection. I have heard it said on more than one occasion when it came to the fall of a famous public leader who had sinned that he had no one to turn to. What is the body of Christ there for? Somehow we must learn as the body (a big family), that it is okay to deal with deeply buried struggles. The truth is, we all have shame about something, and we must bring the issue into the open so that God can cleanse it. He will touch us and remove the blot of our shamefulness as we yield to Him.

Shame is destructive because it causes us to act as if we are children of the light, but secretly we are controlled by forces of darkness. We desperately want freedom but are afraid to trust others. We settle for a life of hidden sin and broken dreams because we never allow our private struggles to come to the surface.

The only way shame can be removed is if it is exposed to the light. Shame is like mold because it grows in the darkness. Once light begins to shine on the shame, that light reveals the truth behind the brokenness and the stain of the shame is removed. Hidden sin only has power over us because we live in secret regarding our struggles.

Once we expose it, the power of the bondage is broken, and it no longer has a grip on us. I have found that when I open up about my secrets, they are not as bad as I thought. I had more fear of the reactions of others toward me than I did about the depth of the pain that the internal darkness was causing in me. The enemy deceives us into believing that if we deal openly with our sins, we will lose our reputation. The truth is that God has delivered us from this lie.

Jesus took upon Himself the shame, our inability to change, upon the cross. He was openly shamed for our sake. The things we hide and the same repetitive weaknesses we have in our life were taken upon the righteous shoulders of Jesus. We can hide them or exchange them. I have learned that bringing light into my darkness brings a great relief of the pressure that has built up over the years. I find peace when I settle these issues with God.

False Belief #5: I've Got to See It to Believe It

There are those who search for signs and those who run from signs. For some of us, if we cannot see God's hand at work in our lives, we give up on believing in Him. We reduce the activity of God in our lives to physical manifestations of His presence. We doubt the promises in the Bible because we see no evidence of them in our lives. As a result, we develop a relationship with our Lord that is rooted in unbelief.

It is odd that we can believe God for big things like our personal salvation and His message of unconditional love, but we struggle to believe He will meet us in our present suffering. If God's position is displaced in our minds, we will live in confusion about His intervention in our lives. God must be the center of our foundation for reality and life. Otherwise, we will look for physical evidence of Him rather than looking to know Him and better understand His nature.

God may be trying to do things in our life that we are not recognizing. Oftentimes we do not view certain incidents as though they were a part of God's plan for us. Yet I have come to realize that God uses everything we go through to teach us and reveal more of Himself to us. We need to be careful that we are not forcing God to move the way we want Him to move. If our frequent cry is, "Answer my prayer, Lord!" but we give up quickly if we do not get an answer right away, we should realize our job is to believe Him and His Word. He will do His part; we must be sure we prepare our hearts to receive His gentle leading.

Unbelief does not move God. However, the enemy thrives when we are skeptical of God's power. If we really want to be free, we must be open to everything God has for us (including the full expression of His gifts in the body of Christ) and utilize the power He has given us to defeat the devil. (See 1 Cor. 12:4–11.) We must let the Holy Spirit flow and wash away our unbelief. The move of the Spirit of God is what brings the supernatural power of God to us. It is for now, not just eternity.

God reveals His plan of restoration, including the outpouring of His Spirit, to each generation. Yet we often corrupt the move of His Spirit by turning it into an issue of personal embellishment. Many groups have made God's Spirit into an idol by worshipping the manifestations of the Spirit rather than God. The Spirit then becomes a thing of possession: "I got my touch from the Holy Spirit; you'd better get yours." The truth is, God sends moves of His Spirit because He mercifully seeks to grow us up in the ways of His kingdom. He continues to add divine revelation to each generation, hoping to bring us into His fullness.

My belief is simple. God's Word is truth. If I will apply that truth to my life by obeying it, then I can expect to receive the fruit of the promises found in His Word. When I struggle to believe, I must go to His Word for strength and encouragement. He speaks to me by His Spirit as I listen to Him. His counsel gives me power to believe.

Hearing His voice in our hearts is all the evidence we need to start the process of seeing His revelation becoming our reality. I have made the mistake in the past of seeking the sign first. No sign follows the revelation; otherwise, Jesus would not have rebuked the Pharisees for seeking a sign (Matt. 12:38–39). Signs are not bad, but if we seek them apart from God, we open ourselves to divination (foretelling future events or receiving hidden information by demonic influences or powers). The Lord gives us signs as an invitation to draw us into a greater reality of His power to save and heal us.

False Beliefs about Others That Prevent Supernatural Transformation

If we are not properly related to God and our perception of self is warped, then our connection with others will be dysfunctional (a sophisticated word for painfully ugly relationships). We form unhealthy relationships because the *goo* in our lives sticks to the *goo* in the lives of others. We cannot just say that we got slimed. We play a role in what we attract and how we relate. Healthy relationships are built on a foundation of love; exchanging that love with one another sets them apart. It can be one of the most rewarding things in the universe to give and receive love, but we must first be willing to receive that love from God our Father. The Father's love sets our relationships in order. The first step is to know God's love for ourselves. If we reverse the order, seeking others to be our foundation for personal security, we get hurt and false beliefs about who we are develop. Let's look at some of them.

False Belief #1: My Life Is a Mess Because Other People Hurt Me

How many times do we have to go around this mountain? We try to find love only to find hurt and more disillusionment. I don't know about you, but I went around that mountain way too many times. I thought I was on the right path and worked hard to play by the rules, only to find it was the same path. The path I am referring to is the one on which relationships that seem so right end up so wrong. I have had my share of dysfunctional associations.

My discoveries about myself during the process of restoration enlightened me in this area of my life. I realized that during all the time I had spent working and doing for God, I had never understood why certain opportunities were sabotaged in my life. Things would seem to be going so well and then something would happen, everything would crumble, and there would be a deep hurt. My way of handling this was to blame. Sometimes I blamed others for my problems (at times I even blamed Satan), and ultimately, I developed a belief that I was a victim.

Have you ever felt like you must have a big V on your chest because you are constantly falling prey to victimization? Victim mentality can form a vicious cycle in our lives. We keep getting set up for the blunt intrusion of other people's sins against us. We don't want to be victimized, but it appears as if we have no control over circumstances. No matter how hard we try to love others, we end up getting hurt by them. This pattern continues until we are worn down. We expect to be hurt in relationships, and what we expect becomes our reality. It doesn't take long before we develop the belief that our purpose in life is to be hurt. We deserve it—so we had better learn how to take it.

I was a mess because of how I chose to deal with the hurt. Everybody gets hurt in relationships. There is no completely safe place to avoid relationship dysfunction. Even the Beav on one of my favorite childhood shows *Leave It to Beaver* experienced emotional trauma. I don't know how he made it growing up in such a perfect family, but we all go through things that are painful—it is how we choose to process that pain that matters.

Granted, some of us have more to work through than others. Some people do grow up in families in which there is gross abuse taking place. I empathize with them. I was in one of those families. There was violence, physical pain, emotional pain, and alcoholism. To this day our family has not been restored, because all of us have not been able to work through the depth of the pain. This pain is dark, evil, and tough to face. But with God's grace, it is possible for us to work through it.

The issue at hand is that many believers excuse themselves from living above their circumstances because they have been hurt, and they spend their lives licking their wounds. Those who live under this "wounded" mentality never allow themselves to become vulnerable; they build relationships founded on the false belief that other people are untrustworthy because of their potential to cause hurt.

A wounded mentality prevents the normal growth of healthy relationships. We can choose to remain victims or begin to trust someone, specifically God. God does not want us to be so reclusive that we form our spirituality in a closet. He gave us a family and others to create an environment of nurture and support.

You may be saying, "You don't know my family." Believe me, I understand what you mean. But we rob ourselves and God of the blessing of fruitfulness if we remain behind closed doors. Trusting others is always a risk, but until we surrender our hurt, we cannot expect a release from it. The strange thing is, even pain can bring emotional comfort. If we spend our days holding onto our pain and allowing it to define our beliefs, we can expect to reap the consequences of a life dominated by bitterness, rejection, and self-hatred.

We will continue to set ourselves up for failure in relationships until we deal with the real problem—our resistance to healing. This resistance stems from a false core belief about life and God. We believe that because other people have hurt us, we deserve to live insulated from the common battles of life. That place does not exist in this world. The battle rages on, regardless of whether or not we choose to fight. It is not a question of whether to fight; it is a question of how to fight. We can sit in our self-pity the rest of our lives, which limits the power of God working in us to transform us, or we can take responsibility for the pain we harbor in our souls and allow God to transform it into something that brings healing for us and others.

Forgiving or not forgiving is not an optional issue in a Christian's life. If we do not forgive, then we cannot be forgiven. These are the clear words of Christ. As a matter of fact, He said that before you worship, you should forgive others (Mark 11:25–26). Paul encouraged the same principle in releasing others before we partake of the Lord's Table. (See 1 Cor. 11:20–34.) All of this is for our benefit as well as for the person who injured us.

Step out of the victim role and into the victor role. Move out of passivity regarding the pain in your soul. Choose to be a forgiver.

Extend grace and mercy to the people in your past, present, and future. It will make a supernatural difference to you.

False Belief #2: I Am Not Okay Unless You Say So

This is the age-old struggle of mankind. We spend our lives seeking the approval of others in order to find personal significance and security. It is hard to understand why we cannot seem to gain the approval of others when we try so hard. Effort is not the issue for most of us. Perception is the problem.

Somewhere along the way, we came to believe that we were unacceptable. This internalization forces the searching for approval to begin.

Yes, it is true some people are hard to please no matter what you do. I remember when I was a young boy, my family required me and my siblings to do work that adults normally did, and we were criticized and shamed if we did not complete the tasks. In my struggle to find acceptance from my family, I formed the belief that unless others approved of me, I was worthless. This deep-seated belief carried over to my relationships in adulthood as I continued my search for acceptance and validation. I was certain that I didn't measure up to others because of my abilities or the lack thereof.

Where is it written that we must have the approval of all of mankind in order to be valuable? This boldface lie was perpetuated by the accuser himself. What happens is, in our striving to find acceptance and security, we fall for the greatest lie of all time: we look to creation to affirm us instead of seeking the approval of our Creator. But value is based upon the inventor's design. Likewise, worth in the eyes of God is based upon the reality that He created us in His image (Gen. 1:26). In addition, He fashioned each one of us with a unique blueprint. That's why I love the saying "God doesn't make junk."

The truth is, the esteem of others will always be fleeting. Approval comes and goes, depending on the mood of the person giving it. People and possessions cannot give you what you need. Only the imprint of the Master Designer guarantees your significance in this world. The choice is yours. You can chase after the approval of others, which may end with a devastating blow of rejection, or you can look into the face of Father God in whose image you were fashioned, and discover your true value.

We all come into this world with a broken image, a crack in our identity. We can search the world over for the right person to mend that crack, but the only One who can fix the broken image is the One who bears the image—God. He fixes our cracked identity by remolding us into the shape He ordained from the foundation of the world. No human being can offer us that impartation.

We increase our security in the Lord as we allow Him to love us. It's that simple. Allowing God's love to fashion our self-image empowers us to connect with others in healthy ways. We can enjoy relationships, giving of ourselves and setting appropriate boundaries, if we base who we are on His loving acceptance.

False Belief #3: Rejection Is My Middle Name

Rejection is ugly and no one deserves it. It is repulsive because it is a lie—it is a judgment of character based on a twisted understanding of our true nature. Here's what happens to cause us to feel rejected. Someone we depend on takes the weakness in our lives and uses it to drive us away. The person throws us away, kicks us to the curb, and is finished with us because we are seen as invaluable. In that person's opinion, we do not have the goods to deserve approval.

How do you respond to such repulsion? The natural inclination of those seeking approval only to be rejected is to consider it deserved. This struggle can lead to a long night in front of the TV, eating a bottomless barrel of rocky road ice cream. But when the medicinal value of the sugar wears off, the reality must be faced. The reality is that you may be at fault and need to deal with that part of your life that is offensive. The other side of the relationship may reveal that the other person who rejected you may have issues. That person is responsible for himself and must place his faults before God.

Recognizing that there are always two parties in relationships and both need to face their selfishness is a good start. If we, the receptors of rejection, walk away believing we deserve to be rejected and thinking that it will only continue, then we have a problem. We invite rejection into our lives if we think we deserve it. Rejection begets rejection. It reproduces after its own kind. The more we allow the cycle to continue, the more it will fashion our character. Others will believe that we deserve it. They will reject us because we take it.

For many of us the problem runs deep, very deep. The reality exists because the course of rejection started in our childhood. Our parents, the ones entrusted with the fragility of our development, rejected us. Their action constitutes a deeply-rooted problem. It does not go away overnight, but the cycle can be broken.

I will address this subject in depth in a later chapter that discusses the healing of wounds, but gaining God's acceptance prepares the way for healing the wounds of rejection. His acceptance works deep down beyond the pain of mere mortals. His embrace and knowing the depth of His love will erase the sting of rejection. The red-hot power of God, speaking into our hearts, is the answer for the word curses others have spoken against us. He created us to pour into us the goodness of His loving embrace. If we look to Him for acceptance, then we can exchange the pain of rejection with His unconditional love for us. This takes place as we practice the principle of receiving His love on a daily basis.

False Belief #4: The Actions of Others Should Not Hurt Me

It is not wrong to be hurt. However, it is ungodly to hold onto that hurt. There is a distortion in the body of Christ regarding how we deal with hurt. Somehow we have acquired the dangerous perception that because we are Christians, we should not be hurt by the harmful actions of others. This pervasive issue is very prominent when it comes to advice given about family relationships. The status quo is to tell people to grin and bear it because that is the moral thing to do.

I don't know about you, but when someone cuts my arm, it bleeds and it hurts. Why should we as Christians act in denial about our pain? There is no scriptural precedent for this. It only perpetuates deep emotional and relational problems. We see the writers of the Psalms coming before others and bellowing out their pain to God. I believe that we are encouraged in the New Testament by Paul and others to bring our grievances to the people who caused them. The only time I do not believe this is healthy is when there is good cause to think the offending party will do further harm.

Our hurts are not going to heal if we deny their existence. Contrary to the old saying "time heals all wounds," it is only by facing the hurts and dealing with the pain that we resolve our offenses. God is in the restoration business, a process that can only begin when we bring everything into the light. He is not the dent doctor who covers everything up and never addresses the real problem. If we are hurt, it is our responsibility to take action. We cannot expect to heal if we keep secret the pain in our souls and our bodies. This is what the substance of the gospel is all about—the process of learning to exchange our pain with His healing.

The power of God comes to those who know they need a doctor, not to those who are too self-reliant to find it or who are participating in a major cover-up. The Lord became a man so that He could identify with our suffering and lift us above it, not so that He could sink into it and give us an excuse to do the same thing. The Lord Jesus Christ overcame all of our sufferings so that we could rise above them with His strength and to His glory.

Exchanging False Beliefs with True Beliefs

I found out that exchanging false beliefs with true ones takes the transforming power of God. While bedridden with hepatitis, I faced the reality of insanity in my own life. Pressed with this life-threatening situation, I was forced to recognize that my beliefs were not working for me. They were not just falling short; they were destroying my life. I came to a very humble place of admission that my core values had driven my body to sickness. This was a defining moment in my life. I quickly realized that if I was going to fully recover, those beliefs had to change.

Gaining discernment was the first step to recovery. I had to discern what lay in darkness in the far reaches of my soul—beliefs which had entered during childhood and were now, in adulthood, eating away all that was good and godly, like a parasite. I turned my life upside down and inside out, looking for the source of problems and the root causes for my fallout. I went against every thread of insecurity in my life. Even though I was afraid of losing control more than the actual experience of death, I opened my life before God and others with complete submission because I was desperate. "Lord, please help me!" was my cry.

I looked into the face of my bewildered wife, which spoke volumes to me. Her struggles were not only a reflection of my leadership but of my sin. My anger, my bitterness, my controlling, my criticism, and my judgmental ways were strangling the life out of her soul. I listened carefully to people around me. Some were close friends and some were casual acquaintances. I went to pastors and leaders within the body of Christ and beseeched them, "Please speak to me about what I'm going through." I begged God for insight and understanding. I was a man on a mission to gain God's Word for my life.

If the cause of my circumstances was hidden sin, as it was with King David when the prophet Nathan addressed him, then I wanted to know. Remember, the prophet told David a story about a rich man who had stolen a poor man's lamb and then killed it to feed a visitor, symbolizing how David had stolen another man's wife and then killed him. Nathan asked David what he would do with that rich man, and without hesitating, David said, "Kill him," to which Nathan replied, "You are the man!" (2 Sam. 12:7). Let me tell you, I know the shear terror of being that man. We all have blind spots, places in our lives in which we are unaware of how we appear to others. The challenge is finding the courage to ask for help. I did, and it saved my life.

We will not experience the deep transforming work of God if we hang onto old habits and beliefs. Letting go of them is a big jump for many people, because the thought of releasing our comforts, props, and protective mechanisms brings fear. People who struggle with addictive or destructive behavior are especially vulnerable to the voice of fear within that says, "Even though this behavior is not working for me, at least I know how to do it."

The process of going through a total transformation—body, soul, and spirit—sounds intimidating and does not come easily. It requires a deep work, which many are not willing to face. It means taking the road less traveled. This path is not comfortable and does not fit into the normal, everyday mindset. Most of us have been conditioned to follow what is popular or safe, or we go for the latest, greatest thing on the market that comes to us in a nice little package without complications and with no hidden costs. The truth is that all change, whether good or bad, is scary. But an even greater truth that should shake us from our comfort zone is that the enemy wants us to remain in darkness, so he will feed us all kinds of lies and temptations in hopes that we sink deeper into his captivity. This is where faith in a Savior who longs to rescue us comes into the picture.

Think about this: How does a capsized ship keep from sinking? Another boat must come alongside and rescue it. A wise captain knows he cannot save his own ship; he must radio for help. The craft must be brought ashore upright, all water must be drained out, and then any damages must be repaired before the ship can ever set sail again. I was a sinking ship. The cracks in my vessel came long before the hull split wide open. The stress fractures were there long before the ship ever started taking on water and sinking. I knew they were there but did not give them any attention. I just kept sailing, believing that I could stay afloat. After all, I was the only one with the ability to captain my ship. Or so I thought.

The truth is, we all need someone to rescue us. Jesus is that someone. He is the only One ever to set sail and overcome the raging sea. It doesn't matter what's wrong or how wrong it is—He has an answer. The quest now is to figure out what is preventing us from receiving His supernatural transformation. He desires that we sail the high seas as valiant sailors, overcoming the rage of the waves in our lives.

It's Time to Get Real!

When I say it's time to get real, I'm not talking about putting on your happy face for friends and family even if you don't feel like it, in an effort to keep your reputation appealing and acceptable. What I am I am saying is, you need to be gut-level, dead-dog, straight-forward, in-your-face real. You must declare an end to the insanity. It has become a matter of life and death.

You cannot afford to miss the life preserver being offered by the rescue ship. Let it all hang out. Quit hiding in the darkness. Hiding prevents the healing process that can only take place in the light. To remain sick as a means of coping with life's difficulties is pure misery and yields a life full of unbelief. People would call us crazy if we were prisoners of war and someone came and unlocked the shackles and prison doors, declaring our freedom, but we chose to remain prisoners. Jesus has freed us. You are free—free to believe and overcome all that "prison life" has done to you.

When I became conscious of the fact that very little good remained in my heart and that I had been living under sick beliefs, I knew I had to rely upon the Holy Spirit to see me through the restoration process. The Holy Spirit has the ability to see the root of our problems— to see what we are not able to see for ourselves. The Counselor, or Helper as He is depicted in the New Testament, then leads us down a gentle path of resolution. This is a process of search and seizure. We must allow God to search our hearts and, as the Spirit leads, to seize those issues that are holding us captive and remove them from our life through deliverance. We cannot move forward if we do not understand what (and whom) we are dealing with, so we will get into that in the next chapter. But wisdom precedes deliverance, and gaining knowledge and wisdom requires time—time with God and time in His Word.

One of the greatest and most subtle attacks the devil has launched on the modern age is to get us to believe that busyness is productivity. The enemy keeps the truth concealed from us because, ironically enough, we are too busy to receive it. He deceives us into believing that we do not have time for the most important thing—developing our intimacy with God.

Time is your most precious commodity. Don't make the mistake I did by squeezing God into planned segments of your life. Make Him the center of your world. An entire generation is at stake, not just your personal restoration. Again I implore you, stop the madness before it is too late. Get real about the beliefs that are the driving force behind your life.

For some, this message will fall upon deaf ears and blind eyes. The enemy has deceived them about the corruption in their life, and they discount this message and the messenger. Don't let that be the case for you. I wish I had paid more attention to what was going on in my life before I crashed. So if you have ears to hear, take heed to my words. Consider them as a divine interruption that could save you from tragedy. I wish someone would have done this for me—given me the plain and simple truth about the path of destruction I was on—before it drove me to illness.

As one of God's messengers of truth, I call you into account. I beg you to stop, search your heart, and determine what you really believe. Take a good, hard look at what (or who) is really driving the ship that you call a life for Christ. If you discover beliefs that do not line up with God's core values, then I hope, by the mercy of God, you will take action to change those beliefs. If you will not take action, then you cannot blame God for the continued failures in your life. It is time to open every door in your life to a fresh change brought about by a just and compassionate God. Now is the time; tomorrow may be too late. So, go ahead—get real with God!

The discipline of God brings correction and ultimately healing, whether it be for an individual or an entire country. One of the problems with us as individuals is that the discipline we received from our parents was so harsh and distorted, we think God is mad at us and is going to give us the same treatment. Yet God disciplines us out of love, not anger, and when He corrects us, it is a part of the plan to restore us, not destroy us. He is seeking to draw us back into His loving arms. Of course, He doesn't cause sickness or other problems in our lives; our struggle with disease and destruction is a symptom of our breaking His natural and spiritual laws. But God can turn the evil in our lives into good as a means of restoring us.

Restoration begins with a seed of truth. That seed grows if it is watered. First, it decomposes and becomes a part of the ground. Then the seedling produces new life as the broken ground fertilizes it. The same process takes place in us. We form our beliefs as we apply truth to our lives. Restoration, or new life, forms as we receive the Word of life. This tiny new plant, if cared for properly, grows into a whole new way of thinking, speaking, and behaving.

God is truth. Make room for Him by dumping the false, ungodly junk. ("Come on back," as they say in the sanitation business.) God will penetrate the layers of darkness with His light. The light of the power of God will break up everything that hinders your receptivity to healing. This may create a crisis for you, but just realize you stand at a crossroad. Yielding to God and following Him down the path of restoration is a process of giving up the control and finding the best, most rewarding life you could ever dream of. That's the God-life. He will patch you up, heal your body, renew your mind, convert your soul, and empower you to become a vessel of His life. Your ongoing relationship with Him will revolutionize your beliefs, and they will become electric. The magnetic power of God will draw you to the point of seeing the impossible become a reality, which will cause your false beliefs to fade like a bad dream.

The past is over; you no longer have to live subject to the old slavery mentality or the taskmaster (Satan) who enslaved you. You can begin right now. Bow down (on your knees or in your heart) before God and repent. Open your mind to change and allow God to clean the house. Let Him do an extreme makeover of your spirit, soul, and body. Exchange the lies for the truth, and ask God to speak into your life.

Prayer:

Father, I come to You, pouring out my heart. I ask for discernment regarding my thoughts toward myself. Help me to

*love myself the way You love me. I want to know Your heart
for my life. I want to reflect You in my thoughts, feelings, and
actions. More than anything, Father, I ask for help to see myself
the way You see me. I ask You to impart to me a deep sense of
my identity in Christ. Let my perception of myself be a positive
and secure one. Likewise, Father, I ask You to help me embrace
others the same way. Father, give me love for others and help me
to extend that love to them even if they do not love me in return.
Let me see the people in my life the way You see them. Give me
supernatural love and strength to reach out to others and affirm
them. Help me, Lord, to love others the way I want to be loved.
In the name of Jesus. Amen.*

CHAPTER 5

THE REAL WAR OF TRANSFORMATION, PART 1

The Battle for Our Soul

WHETHER OR NOT WE LIKE IT OR WANT TO ADMIT IT, there is a kingdom of darkness that exists and in very real ways can show up in our lives. We see it around us every day, and we know by discernment that evil exists. Yet there is an enormous distortion of truth regarding the spirit world, largely because of the way it has been illustrated by the media. They have used the presence of darkness to entertain us within the context of scary movies, dreadful talk shows, and "reality" TV, and they make a mockery of the powers of darkness as if the spiritual battle were a game show we can simply turn off and on at will. These freaky demonstrations of extreme vulgarity are no longer out of the ordinary but have become commonplace in the entertainment industry. Although many of us would quickly herald that we do not participate in such levels of grossness, some of us are unaware of the ways in which we do.

For instance, in my own life I would not have linked my struggle with anxiety to the stronghold of demonic fear and the generational pattern of dread that were handed down to me inherently by my parents. But when I approached these deep-seated fears as though I were in an emotional struggle and a spiritual battle, I made great progress. Once my eyes were opened to the presence of the enemy who taunted me daily with various fears, I was better able to tear down my ungodly beliefs and overcome the fear in my life. My point is that we brush off the nonsense of Hollywood and view it as moral bankruptcy, yet we overlook the obvious struggles with evil, like fear, in our own lives.

Though we might like to believe there is no evil in our lives, we must understand that there is an individual who wars against the salvation of mankind. The devil, or Satan, adamantly opposes our transformation by the power of the Holy Spirit. Nothing intimidates Satan more than we who come back from the grave (spiritually speaking), for *self* and the *will of the flesh* have been crucified with Christ (Gal. 2:20). We who walk in newness of life are no longer governed by our earthly nature, but now we have submitted ourselves to another—the risen Lord and Savior. As transformed men and women, by our new nature, we incite the declaration of war because our enemy knows that we are unstoppable—unless we are deceived into thinking otherwise.

I know from experience that when we begin to use terms such as *Satan, the devil, demon, deliver,* or *deliverance,* many people become frightened or turned-off, or they start gazing into our eyes, looking for signs of psychosis. Dealing with the devil creates discomfort for most of us, ministers included, mainly because we don't have training on how to deal with evil. It is hard for us to connect our emotional and physical struggles with the unseen world around us. We may know intuitively that the prince of the air can influence us, but to what degree is another subject we would rather not discuss. Yet to be transformed, we need to know our enemy and how to deal with him.

Scripture teaches that we are to be separate from the world and its evil influence (2 Cor. 6:17). That is the challenge before us. Some say that in order to separate ourselves from evil, we must eliminate every worldly form of evil we can. They feel that if television, radio, computers, or contact with the general public open us up to the world's system, then we are not to use these means of technology or go out and mingle with the worldly population. Others say those mediums in themselves are not inherently evil, but how and why we use them make them evil. So these people have a very open policy and try to sanctify the world's system. The approach Jesus took was that it is not what's on the outside that makes us unclean or full of evil but what emanates from our heart. Getting evil out is not about simply removing every temptation or avoiding becoming one with the world; it is about learning who we are in Christ and living like we are children of our heavenly Father.

I am not setting myself up as the authority on the demonic realm. My desire is to empower any believers who do not understand how they were taken captive by the enemy to find God's freedom from the presence of evil. Most people have not witnessed a balanced, healthy approach to deliverance from demonic oppression as an act of love. I am not advocating that the only means for healing and spiritual growth is the disarming of the devil in the lives of hurting people through deliverance ministry, nor do I believe that all mankind's problems are simply the work of the devil or that there is a demon behind every bush. My recognition is much different: as free moral agents, we are given the choice either to submit to God or to surrender to the oppressive pursuit of the enemy. The beliefs formed as a result of the oppressive work of Satan are the most crucial elements of destruction, and they must be recognized and replaced with the truth of God's Word.

I believe people have a distaste for the subject of deliverance ministry because of how inappropriately it has been used by a few ministers whose attitude is excessively aggressive and condemning toward those who are searching for answers to their problems. Consequently, innocent, hurting people, whose end lies in the wake of condemnation, have become the battleground. When the tools of God's kingdom are abused, people get hurt. That is not at all what Christ died for.

Deliverance ultimately affects the future of the church because there are multitudes of desperate and bewildered people knocking on our church doors who can be helped through deliverance prayer. So the church is left with a choice: to take action or live in denial. I know of and have personally experienced the healthy process of deliverance in other ministries. It can be done the right way—to God's glory and for the freedom of those who are bound.

If you think about it, the overall story of the triumph of the human race is about the battle between good and evil. The consistent theme of the Bible is about how good, represented by God, clashes with evil, represented by Satan. The stage for this inevitable war is set as we daily declare our allegiance to either good or evil. Joshua said it this way: "Choose this day whom you will serve" (Josh. 24:15). The only way to choose correctly is to be informed about the choices. We've been talking about the Lord; now we're going to look closer at His enemy, the enemy of our soul.

Our Real Enemy

The apostle Paul said, "We do not wrestle against flesh and blood, but against principalities, against powers, against the world's rulers, of the darkness of this age, against spiritual wickedness in high places" (Eph. 6:12). For him to say we do not wrestle with real flesh and blood makes it clear that people are not our enemies; there are greater forces for which we must account. Our real enemy is the devil. It is against Satan and his invisible kingdom of demonic spirits that we fight.

The first question we must tackle is, "Are Satan and evil spirits real?" This debatable issue has been minimized with the advent of modern science. Our world bases truth on what can or cannot be measured with scientific skill. If it cannot be proven under a microscope, it is not real. Yet professionals who use the sciences to explain the world know that there are certain elements of the material world that are unexplainable. The scientific method does not apply to observing the spiritual realm of the forces of darkness and light. Christians base their faith on the unseen force of a Savior most have never seen.

According to the Bible, Satan and his demons are real and active, especially in their mission to harass believers. You may disagree, but my experience tells me that it is true. So I am going to use not only the sacred writings of scripture, but also my undeniable personal experience; I will be sharing scriptural truth on this subject in the context of what has worked in my own life.

I experienced the reality of confronting demons when I was attacked in my flesh and became so sick. The greatest revelation God gave me about my illness, which also happened to be a very shocking discovery, was that I had partnered with evil to get that way. On my journey to find healing, I discovered that my behavior had opened the door to the presence of evil. In a previous chapter, we learned that our choices are motivated by our core beliefs. That is precisely what created the opportunity for me to be taken captive by the enemy. I brought this on myself!

Facing my coexistence with evil was much more difficult than hearing the diagnosis of hepatitis. Nevertheless, although there was a fierce reckoning that came with exposure to the true condition of my soul, I was able to handle it appropriately, and it caused me to become utterly broken and humbled before God—setting me up to encounter His deep redemptive love.

On my journey toward healing, I discovered while trudging through the soil of my soul that my condition was not only physical, but also connected to my spiritual and emotional problems. Remember, we are body, soul, and spirit, and the strength or weakness of one will affect the other two. First, I was affecting my health by breaking God's natural laws through eating and resting improperly. I thought I was invincible. I ran on caffeine and sugar, and stayed up late watching television each night, as many people do. Secondly, I violated the commandments of Christ because I was holding bitterness toward others who had hurt me. I carried that hurt, internalized it, and allowed it to fester. I pushed it so deep into the recesses of my soul that I did not realize it was still there. Thirdly, I was in rebellion toward God. I decided I was going to run my life, family, and ministry my way, with good Christian intentions, of course—and we've already seen what's wrong with that kind of "I'm-in-charge" lifestyle.

At first glance there seems to be no out-of-the-ordinary presence of evil in the description of my decline. We all struggle with lifestyle issues—the battle for some may be with eating, for others it may be work habits, and for a number of people it may be self-esteem related to our relationships. Where's the evil? Most of us probably would say that to consider those normal struggles to be rooted in evil is ludicrous or at least fanatical. So let's go deeper into my case study.

Some have questioned me as to how this curve of illness in my life could happen when I was doing the work of the Lord. The reason is that I was striving with anger, which led me right into Satan's trap. I was so enraged about the course of my life that I was blind to the obvious assault of the adversary on my family and me. I was bent on proving that my way was superior to the way taken by those who had hurt me, and I was even hurling accusations at God. It was full-blown rebellion, not just "righteous indignation" or a case of "working through my issues." My anger was fueled by the utter despair in my soul, which was screaming at me for wasting some of the best years of my life, helping a man build his kingdom only to see it ultimately come crashing down.

All I could think of was that I was a puppet for the church. I was filled with self-hatred, which was fueled by the voice of the devil who screamed at me daily about how worthless I was. The real trouble was that I accepted his lies and put them into action as if they were reality. Remember, anytime I could stand it, I drowned my sorrows in activity (good works), alcohol, junk food, ungodly entertainment, and anything else that would afford me the opportunity to escape my misery. Being a servant of God does not give us immunity from the works of the enemy if we are walking in darkness.

When our bodies become exhausted, we are prime candidates for burnout, viruses, chronic fatigue, and a host of other physical struggles that stem from a compromised immune system. We get sick because our bodies are subject to emotional, physical, and spiritual things that do not belong in our systems. My disobedience brought pressure and anxiety; I was living a lie, which exposed me to great stress. Stress comes from getting living out of line with God's created order, the way He set things up for us. It takes a lot of energy to live in opposition to God's divine order; my lowered energy levels exposed my body to weakness, and I became a prime candidate for disease and sickness. The devil did not just walk up to me and fling a deadly virus on me. No, over time, I took the bait and fell for his lies, which caused me to wear out and become weak.

That's how the enemy works. He picks out the one in the flock who is limping and targets that person for attack. Is that fair? Nothing is fair when it comes to war, and it did not take long for me to realize that I was in a war for my life. I don't know of any other leaders in the church I was working for who became ill. As far as I know, I was the only one. I believe the reason it happened to me was the way I responded to the situation. I had a choice to make: I could sit around and feel sorry for myself, which would only make matters worse, or I could go to God and repent and deal with the matter through His supernatural love. I got a revelation during this time that the answer to my problems was not at the bottom of the pit. I knew I dug the hole and I knew it was plenty deep. I could keep digging like that was going to get me somewhere, or I could look up and cry out for help.

The point is, I didn't find the answer by dissecting everything that was bad about me. That is what I call worm theology: "I am just a worm trying to crawl through life." No, I needed someone to reach into my pit, grab my hand, and lift me to safety . . . and then take my shovel and use it on my backside, as my grandmother would say.

My battle with illness was actually about learning how to repossess what I had unknowingly given up to the enemy. I do not believe Satan has the power to just make us sick at will. He must be given access to our life. I threw open the door to him with my sin.

Sin is more than missing the mark. Our sin leads us away from the Father, our protection. It separates us from God. The separation is what the enemy used to divide me from my protector. My guard was down—I was too busy with my hand to the plow, "working for God," to see my enemy approaching. I did not see him coming because I was blind with rebellion and anger. I was struggling with addictions, striving with my wife and family, running on anxiety, bitter at the church and several other people, and holding a ransom over my own head that read, "Fix these problems or else." I was very easy prey.

Who's Running the Show?

If we are going to find the answers to our struggles, our discernment must increase. Discernment comes from hanging out in the light. We cannot just take a laissez-faire approach to life and expect everything to work out in our favor. All of us are subject to the subtle approach of the enemy because we live in a physical world that is governed from a spiritual dominion. The ordinary affairs of our lives are subject to the spiritual conflict taking place in our souls. So we must be careful—normal is not just normal.

If we look at the course of a day as a set of normal occurrences that are the result of human will and the forces of nature, we stand to miss the deeper side of life. The enemy of our soul, Satan, can influence the course of events in our lives through our thoughts. He approaches us with an idea, hoping to get us to absorb it and put it into play. If the devil influences our decisions, he succeeds; then his kingdom and rule advance in our lives.

I teach this concept across the country and some people doubt it. They believe that teaching about the devil only gives him power. But the fact is, he already has power. Adam gave him dominion and power in the earth when Adam disobeyed God and ate of the forbidden tree (Gen. 2:16–17; 3:6). Others feel that to teach about Satan is to deify him over Christ. Yet that already happens in the lives of those (Christians included) who have an idolatrous affair with the material world. The enemy may not necessarily be purposefully deified in our lives; nevertheless, he can run the show when we let him.

Not teaching people about the power of darkness is creating a vicious cycle within the walls of the church. Multitudes of people live and die in torment as certified members of local churches. My experience has taught me that Satan and his cohorts are presently active, seeking to bring destruction to the lives of believers and nonbelievers alike. The sad thing is, we give him the power because we are not aware of his presence nor do we know how to defend ourselves from his lies.

You don't need to accept my experience alone as proof. The reality of Satan's existence is an indisputable fact in the Bible. The first followers of Christ watched Him cast out devils to free those in bondage, listened to demons scream at the very glimpse of His presence, saw Him heal the sick by casting out devils, and observed Him go face-to-face with the devil to emerge as the victorious King over all principalities. In case you want further proof, let's take a look at some scriptures that teach us about the enemy.

The apostle Paul talked about being hindered by Satan (1 Thess. 2:18). Peter warned us how Satan walks around like a roaring lion, seeking someone he may devour (1 Peter 5:8). James urged believers to submit to God and resist the devil in order to make him flee (James 4:7). John addressed the seven churches in his prophetic revelations, speaking openly about the work of the devil among first century believers. (See Rev. 2.) Even Christ had a face-to-face encounter with the devil in the wilderness (Matt. 4:1–11), and before Jesus' crucifixion, He said that the adversary came for Him but had no place in Him (John 8:37–44).

The central message of the gospel of Jesus Christ is about the installation of His Father's kingdom here on earth in the lives of His people. Jesus spent His life teaching and equipping His disciples to believe and follow His example. He made it very clear that there is an opposing kingdom that must be removed in order for His to be established. The kingdom of darkness is held in place on earth by the people who indulge in the pleasures of this world and by the religious who live in denial about the existence of this real empire of evil.

Jesus knew of the devil's existence before the world began and spoke of it in Luke 10:18 when He said, "I saw Satan fall from Heaven like lightning." One of the early experiences of Christ's public ministry started with deliverance of demons (Mark 1:23–27), and some of His final instructions to His disciples concluded with coaching about the devil (Mark 16:15–18). Before Jesus ministered to people publicly, He met the enemy face-to-face, setting in order the corruption of man by the first Adam (Matt. 4:1–11; Rom. 5:10–21; 1 Cor. 15:45–58). As you can see, the subject of the two kingdoms was paramount to Christ.

Did Jesus believe in a literal devil and demons? The credibility of His teachings on any subject must be doubted if His teachings and actions regarding the devil were mythical. If He alluded to face-to-face encounters with a mythical figure and cast out imaginary spirit beings, then who is to say He was not referring to a mythical salvation for the souls of mankind? The beloved apostle John told us that the reason the Son of God appeared was to destroy the devil's work (1 John 3:8 KJV). So, yes, Jesus Christ of Nazareth not only believed in a literal devil, He dethroned him and will ultimately destroy him. This is not a cosmic pretend battle but a real epic that will be unfolded before our very eyes with or without our participation.

There's no denying these biblical truths: Jesus was serious about believing in the existence of a personal devil, Jesus came to dethrone Satan from His kingdom, Jesus cast real evil spirits out of the souls of real people, and Jesus had a face-to-face encounter with the tempter in the wilderness. If this is not enough evidence, here are seven specific New Testament accounts when Jesus cast devils out of certain people:

1. The man in the synagogue tormented by an unclean spirit in Mark 1:21–28 and Luke 4:31–37

2. The blind and mute demoniac in Matt. 12:22–29, Mark 3:22–27, and Luke 11:14–26

3.   The Gergesenes demoniacs in Matt 8:28–34 and Mark 5:1–20; and the Gadarenes demoniac in Luke 8:26–39

4.   The Syrophoenician woman's daughter in Matt. 15:21–28 and Mark 7:24–30

5.   The epileptic boy in Matt. 17:14–21, Mark 9:14–29, and Luke 9:37–43

6.   The woman with a spirit of infirmity in Luke 13:10–17

7.   The mute demoniac in Matt. 9:32–34

The number of instances of deliverance in the New Testament alone indicates the importance of deliverance as a tool of ministry.

Upon His ascension to heaven, Jesus instructed His disciples to advance His kingdom, including casting out demonic spirits (Mark 16:17). The early church was summoned by Christ to follow in His footsteps, be filled with the power of the Holy Spirit, preach the Good News of Christ, and demonstrate His power by healing the sick and casting out evil spirits. As you can see, none of this is new information; it is actually traditional teaching of the early church. Wouldn't you agree that the foundation of the first church was built on the reality of knowing the significance of the unseen world?

The reformation of the modern-day church weighs in the balance as men of God debate the reality of their "celestial enemy." A move of God is sweeping the earth, awakening believers to the real conflict between light and darkness. When the church rediscovers the active power of the Holy Spirit and unleashes it, the whole world will see that God is not powerless, but just waiting for us to take our position of authority over our archrival, Satan.

The Left-Brain Dilemma

The left hemisphere of the brain is the rational side that bases fact on logic. Most of us have a logical side. It can hinder the awareness of spiritual discernment because we are looking for the facts to support the intuition about evil. I ran into this when I was sick. One of my main problems was that my psychological training had given ample rational ammunition to discredit the real presence of my adversary. So I thought I had become too smart to become prey to the devil. There was a time when I believed that he or one of his minions could pressure me, but I had grown to believe that it was rationally impossible now. The Word of God says, "Pride goes . . . before a fall" (Prov. 16:18). I was so prideful that I was taken captive in my spiritual arrogance and ignorance—and it almost cost me my life.

Before this happened, I had reasoned that the concern with evil spirits and the spiritual practices of dealing with devils was only for the fanatical. I had allowed myself to be deceived by the beliefs of Western Christian thinking with regard to the powers of darkness. I was leaning very hard upon the educational training that I received, which minimized the presence of real demonic forces. I learned the hard way that ignorance about Satan is not bliss.

Christian counseling can be credible and effective. I truly believe the modern approach of counseling has served to help many people who suffer from emotional troubles. Remember, I started my journey by going to a Christian counselor. The valuable advice I received then and also at various points along the way enhanced my healing process.

Nonetheless, I would like to point out that the infiltration of secularization within the Christian counseling industry has created more of a clinical atmosphere than a spiritual one in many cases. Counselors who lean solely on the left-brain process miss opportunities to discern the work of a deeper spiritual activity in the life of a counselee. Sometimes the textbook approach to neurosis, which is limited to cognitive restructuring, must be thrown out and the Holy Spirit invited into the healing process. In order to help people who are suffering from both mental and spiritual torment, the spiritual element must be addressed and a valid spiritual remedy offered.

If we are looking for a predominantly scientific explanation for why we choose to collaborate with evil, then we will minimize our actions, writing them off as "human behavior." In the same way, if we observe human behavior and try to analyze it logically, we will limit ourselves. The human spirit has intuitive radar that detects what is going on in the spirit realm. I don't know how many times my wife has said to me when she meets someone who has questionable character that there is something fishy about the person. Her correctness is remarkably precise because her discernment is God-given. This spiritual insight is not computable by experimental or behavioral science, yet our track record with the people in question verifies her accuracy.

Generally, people groups in third world nations acknowledge the spirit world's influence on human behavior without question. Many missionaries report a widespread receptiveness to deliverance ministry in foreign countries. These missionaries say that the effectiveness and ability of ministries overseas is deeper and richer than it is in America because people in countries abroad do not have mental blocks preventing openness to the spirit world as we do in the United States.

The American gospel is typically a promotion of conservative morality, which is given as a remedy for human struggles. The gospel is taught as a model lifestyle. Key moral issues are reinforced with the expectation that people will conform to the standards of Christian morality. This is a good thing, but it is incomplete. Unless we are equipped with the power to overcome the root problem of all immorality (sin), we become exhausted trying to perform the righteous lifestyle. The fact is that our awareness of immorality does not empower us to overcome it.

It's the old deer-in-the-headlights scenario. He sees the lights coming, but instead of moving and escaping danger, he walks right into it. I find that we can cover up spiritual strongholds with good morality and call it Christianity. Publicly we renounce ungodly behaviors, but privately, all too often, we fall prey to them. Where is the power in the American gospel? It's obvious that something is missing. That something is more than rational, left-brained thinking; it is the raw power of God to save, heal, and deliver His people—and it is our only hope in the fight against spiritual realities.

The force of evil is not eliminated because we hold certain truths to be our standards. Evil is something we cannot overcome by universal peace and good will. Evil is demonic at its core and is too great for us to overcome by human standards. The whole purpose for the birth, death, and resurrection of Christ was to overcome evil and thereby establish the kingdom of God in the hearts of men. Evil cannot be overcome through the teaching of moral and ethical values, but by the power of God given to us through the Holy Spirit. Through healing prayer and prayers of deliverance, we become instruments for Jesus to heal and deliver individuals, communities, and institutions from evil.

The Ostrich Syndrome

Are you beginning to see the reality of Satan or are you denying his existence? Denial is a place of false security created by the enemy himself. Some people feel safer in denial; they have what I call the "ostrich syndrome." When an ostrich sticks its head in the sand, its entire body is left completely exposed and vulnerable. Get the picture? While we are retreating from the enemy, hoping he will never show up, he is plotting a surprise attack on our lives. Our adversary has two main jobs: to keep the lost in blindness and to keep Christians in deception. Denial is a form of deception. Deception is the trick of the enemy to lure us into a state of passivity regarding his tactics, which involve our destruction.

If we refuse to face the reality of the presence of darkness that influences our lives, we run the risk of being taken captive by the enemy. Paul warned Timothy, his spiritual son, to be careful regarding the evil one because he seeks to capture those who are in opposition to God (2 Tim. 2:24–26). Just because we have a well-refined rationalization regarding why evil has no influence over our lives does not mean the devil does not exist or that his plan to destroy us is put on hold. I have heard it said that if we do not feel the heat of the spiritual battle, maybe it is because we are running in stride with the adversary himself.

The only way to win the spiritual battles with our adversary is to face him and remove him from our lives with the spiritual authority given to us by God in Christ Jesus. Have you ever ignored a physical problem like an ache or a sore on your body? The pain does not just go away. The malady gets worse if there is no intervention. Likewise, if you choose to stick your head in the sand and try to hide from evil, you'd better be careful; it may bite you in the "pew cushion." Be reminded that when Jesus overcame the devil in the wilderness, the scripture indicates that the tempter departed from Him *for a season* (Luke 4:13). Note that if the devil did not give up on our Lord, who is to say he will give up on us just because we play the game as if he does not exist? As a matter of fact, Jesus said in His teachings to the disciples in the Sermon on the Mount that they should expect to be persecuted for righteousness (Matt. 5:10–12). The point is that Christ was attacked for His stand on righteousness and, as His followers, we will be attacked also. We can either run from the devil or face him with the power of God. The choice is ours to make.

I invite you to get your head out of the sand! Take the place appointed to you by God before the foundation of the earth. We have an appointed position, a place of great significance in this war between the two kingdoms of light and darkness. Our battle cry is, "By the blood of Christ I am a son/daughter of the Most High God, and I stand representing His light, His love, and His life. No weapon formed against me shall prosper nor deter me from my inheritance in Christ. I will overcome by the word of my testimony and by the blood of the Lamb."

We must fight the enemy if we expect transformation of the soul and health to the body. The body itself is designed to fight. The immune system is able to annihilate rogue cells every day if equipped with proper nutrition. There is a constant balancing effort going on within our bodies, bringing homeostasis (stability and equilibrium) to our internal systems. All enemies are quickly extinguished and eliminated. The body has a no-tolerance policy. If we put something toxic in our system, the body is quick to dissolve it and eliminate it. We must develop the same posture in our spiritual life.

We cannot expect the spiritual war penetrating our souls to vanish because we fill our days with busyness and human productivity. We must learn how to engage in spiritual war against the enemy of our souls. I will show you how in the next chapter.

The frontline of battle is calling our name. We must engage and fight. This will not go away. The distant sound of the bomb shells of the enemy are closer than we want to admit. Make your battle plan and get heaven's strategy. Fight! Fight! Fight!

Prayer:

Father God, I run to You! I seek Your heart for the freedom of my soul. Only You can set me free. I have been taken captive. I recognize the enemy's advance in my life and I repent. Give me discernment. Increase my revelation of who You are. Deliver me from evil. I want all evil out of my life. Search my heart. Show me where I have allowed the enemy's strongholds to build up in my life. Bring me out of darkness and into the light. You are the only One who can empower me to be free. I ask in the name of Jesus Christ that the power of darkness be broken in my life. Give me rest in Your strength, for You are my shelter and my strong tower against my foe. Thank You, Father, for victory. Thank You for sending Jesus to spoil the plans of my enemy, Satan. Lord, You are victorious, and I stand ready to receive complete victory in my life. Thank You, Jesus, for defeating Satan and rendering him powerless. And thank You for protecting me. Glory to the risen Lamb! Amen.

CHAPTER 6

THE REAL WAR OF TRANSFORMATION, PART 2

The Weapons of Our Warfare

COMING TO THE REALIZATION THAT WE ARE UNDER THE influence of evil and actually fighting against it are two different things. We need divine power to win the battle against our enemy. Human strength is inadequate; we cannot fight against him on our own. We are no match for the evil one, even on our best day. The power and authority to fight Satan must come from God. Remember, James said, "Submit yourselves to God. Resist the devil, and he will flee from you" (James 4:7). If you recall, submission to God involves learning to yield our will to the Lord every day, one hour at a time.

Yielding to God empowers us to receive a new identity based on relationship with Christ, our Messiah. We yield by emptying our lives of self and filling our lives with His presence. Having His presence in us establishes our authority. It all comes down to whom we know and by whom we are known. His shadow over our lives creates a place of safety and refuge from our enemy (Ps. 91:1–3). In that place of shelter, we are secure, knowing in our hearts that we have already won because Jesus defeated our adversary at the cross.

God commissions us to battle, just as the armed forces commissions recruits. A new recruit who joins a military branch in the United States is informed during his basic training that his number one priority is to remember for whom he is fighting—and the soldier puts his life on the line to protect the honor of God and country. Every ounce of his being is trained to yield complete allegiance to the commander in chief. When we become born again, we are enlisted in the body of Christ for the same purpose. We are called to lay down our lives for the Captain of our salvation (Luke 9:23–24; Heb. 2:10), but we cannot expect to walk in authority without having first surrendered to it. If we desire to win complete victory at all costs, we must first surrender our complete allegiance to our Commander in Chief, Jesus Christ. He shall lead us into battle for His name's sake.

The preservation of our lives and the advancement of God's kingdom are proportional to our yielding to the Commander in Chief of this spiritual war. He is the power and strength and authority, and He alone enables us to win this conflict. All orders and deferment of power come directly from God Almighty Himself. If we submit to Him, He guarantees our protection and freedom as His beloved sons and daughters. But this doesn't mean that we will not experience the dust, smoke, and conflict of the battle. Soldiers go through battle and there is the possibility of bloodshed. It is no different in spiritual warfare.

God promises to meet us as we fight, not as we seek to avoid the battle altogether—and He has given us spiritual weapons to use in combat. In fact, the resources at the disposal of the believer are many. The focus of this chapter will be on those weapons and tools that equip believers to take back their health, their freedom, their finances, their families, their lives. We will be looking at the two categories scripture gives us to establish the strength of the believer in this war: (1) the identity of a believer, and (2) the resources (weapons) used for launching an offense and setting up a defense against the enemy.

The Armor of God

The basis for the foundation of warfare is found in Ephesians 6:12–18, a passage in which Paul portrays his example of how the godly armor of a Christian soldier is used to extinguish the fiery darts of the enemy. In this passage, the identity of a believer is based upon the belt of truth, the breastplate of righteousness, the gospel shoes of peace, the shield of faith, the helmet of salvation, the sword or the Word of God, and prayer that includes praying in the Spirit. Each component fortifies the believer to walk in victory.

The armor is like every other aspect of God's provision—it must be appropriated. Each piece of armor must be used and applied if we expect to see victory. The armor does not fight the battle for us; we must assume our position, practice using our weapons, and learn our commands. A savvy soldier always enters into battle prepared. So we're going to look at each piece of equipment and discuss how to use it. Let's begin with the first one that Paul mentions.

Belt of Truth

Truth is what holds all of the other pieces of armor in place. The belt of truth is the first piece of equipment Paul talks about, because the body of armor is unified by truth (Eph. 6:14). It is interesting to note that the enemy's very first attack against mankind centered on the issue of truth: when Satan spoke to Eve in the garden, he challenged the truth of God's Word, and she fell for his lie (Gen. 3:1–6). From her example, we can see how important it is to know what God has said and is saying. It is His truth that extinguishes every lie of the enemy.

Truth comes from knowing God's Word as a present reality (John 17:17). The Word only has power if we know how to use it. Memorizing scripture is a good thing, but we need more than head knowledge if we want to overcome temptation—the Word must be alive in our hearts. Jesus did not just quote Old Testament scripture to the devil when He was confronted by the evil one in the desert (Matt. 4:1–11). No, Jesus spoke truth that flowed from His convictions about the Father's established kingdom on earth. Jesus hurled the Word at the enemy, and there was no comeback on the part of the devil; he was forced to retreat.

Breastplate of Righteousness

The second part of identity for the believer is the weapon of righteousness, which resembles a breastplate (Eph. 6:14). In Bible days, the breastplate of a Roman soldier was made up of two parts: one covered the vital organs from neck to thighs in the front, and the other covered the back area, thereby serving as a protective covering for the most vulnerable parts of the body. The Roman breastplate is a great illustration of what the righteousness of God is to believers. I like the way Albert Barnes describes it in his Bible commentary: "The idea here may be that the integrity of life, and righteousness of character, is as necessary to defend us from the assaults of Satan, as the coat of mail [or the breastplate] was to preserve the heart from the arrows of an enemy."[1]

Righteousness is imputed, or given, to us by our relationship with God through Christ (Rom. 3:22). The cleansing and depth of His work in our lives is dependent upon our direct appropriation of this gift of righteousness. As soldiers of God, we are good enough, not because of might or skill but because we receive and wear this breastplate that is fashioned for us in righteousness.

How often does the enemy come against us and try to disqualify us because of our struggle with repetitive sin? The fear of being separated from God because we feel we don't measure up can drive us out of His presence and into the enemy's hands. That's the devil's tactic—trying to make us think we don't measure up so that we spend our lives striving to measure up.

We must always keep in mind that our righteousness comes through Jesus and Jesus alone. We are sons and daughters before God, our Father, because Jesus made a way for that relationship. Now life is about learning how to be a faithful son (or a daughter), not wondering if we are one.

Gospel Shoes of Peace

The third component is the message of peace, symbolized in the form of shoes for the feet. Having our "feet shod with the preparation of the gospel of peace" (Eph. 6:15) is not referring to actual shoes, but to being prepared to carry the gospel of peace and be messengers of good tidings.[2] Among the armor of Roman soldiers were military shoes, which were a type of sandal "bound by thongs over the instep and round the ankle, and having the soles thickly studded with nails."[3] The Greek word for this type of shoe translates "readiness" and is sometimes used in the sense of "establishment," "firm foundation," or "firm footing."[4]

A soldier whose feet are strong can climb any obstacle when waging war against the enemy. The "readiness shoe" assured the soldier of a sure foundation upon which to stand, just as the gospel of Jesus Christ assures believers their foundation in Him is solid. We are able to stand constantly and firmly in the faith of the gospel, and so strive and contend for it without being moved from it.[5]

A soldier whose feet are tired and sore cannot stand to fight. The battle is given to those who can stand against the enemy. Peace gives great strength because, in the face of the storms of battle, the soldier knows he is going to win. A soldier who knows his destiny has peace, and that good news will carry him to victory.

I am amazed that Jesus—with perfect peace in His heart—performed miracles among His rivals who were looking to kill Him. Notice that Jesus did not have to strive to do miracles; He said He was only doing what He had seen the Father doing (John 8:28). The invitation is powerful—peace comes from obedience. The bottom line is, our feet will carry us along a path that either produces strife and anxiety or yields peace and power.

Shield of Faith

The fourth piece of armor, the shield of faith, alludes to our building a strong identity in Christ (Eph. 6:16). Good soldiers recognize the attack of their enemy, and they are skilled in shielding themselves during the onslaught. In spiritual warfare, we fight using faith as our shield: when the enemy launches thoughts of unbelief, we rise up in faith (in the inner man), extinguishing those fiery darts of doubt. As soldiers, we remember the orders of our Commander in Chief and rise to defend ourselves in victory.

The night Jesus was betrayed, He warned His disciples to pray so that they would not fall into temptation (Matt. 26:41–43). But instead of praying, they all fell asleep. He, on the other hand, waited before God and exchanged His will with the will of the Father. For that reason, Jesus was able to give away His life for the sins of the world, which was the greatest demonstration of faith ever produced by a human being.

We must not fall asleep during the heat of battle. Our goal should be to learn to use our faith as a weapon to extinguish the lies (the darts) of the enemy and to believe God for a role in establishing His kingdom here on earth.

Helmet of Salvation

The helmet of salvation, our fifth piece of armor, protects our thinking (Eph. 6:17). Why do our minds need protection from the enemy? In 2 Corinthians 11:3, Paul warned the Corinthian church to be careful lest they be deceived by the serpent and forget the simplicity of the gospel and their pure devotion to Christ. This passage suggests that deception takes place in our mind—that part of us where reasoning, remembering, and forgetting occur. As soldiers in God's army, we must also realize that our mental outlook greatly affects our ability to execute God's plan on the battlefield; much of the battle is either won or lost in our minds. In addition, the pulling down of strongholds (a stronghold is the place where the enemy sets up his access to our thinking; 2 Cor. 10:4), which Paul talks about, takes place in the mind.

Keeping God's protective helmet in place begins with understanding salvation: "Salvation, the consciousness that we have a Savior 'able to save unto the uttermost,' gives the Christian soldier courage for the conflict."[6] Salvation promotes confidence and the means to pull down the enemy's strongholds because it reassures the warrior he is protected. If we know we are winning a battle, we fight altogether differently than if we question the outcome. Salvation by grace, the impartation of divine favor, empowers us to fight as winners.

Don't let Satan into your head. He only has the power to question salvation, not take it away. Keep your mind focused on the truth (the Word), and you will finish strong in the race that is set before you.

Sword of the Spirit—the Word of God

The previous weapons are used to protect; this component of armor is the weapon used to assail the enemy (Eph. 6:17). The Bible is not the physical sword of a soldier in a nation's army. God's sword is the sword of the Spirit, which is the Word of God. Many of God's soldiers make the mistake of slinging the words of the Bible in the face of the devil to no avail. The successful combatant receives the Word of God, made active by the Spirit of God, and then uses those words as a sword to defeat the adversary. The Word of God does not have power unless we receive it by faith and allow the Holy Spirit to activate it in our lives.

Many Christians are defeated when trying to use the Word of God because they approach it as a requirement of God that they must do themselves. That is legalism. You cannot fulfill the Word without the Spirit. That is why Jesus gave us both. He even said it is better for us that He left earth for our sake so that the Spirit would come to empower us to overcome (John 16:7). Otherwise, the Word is another law that man cannot fulfill on his own.

Prayer and Praying in the Spirit

Prayer is considered by many biblical scholars to be Paul's final weapon of warfare. It is to be used in conjunction with our armor for victory in spiritual battles. In Paul's day it was customary for the Greek armies, before they went into battle, to offer prayers to their gods for success. Paul was showing us in Ephesians 6:18 that we, as spiritual warriors, must depend on the Captain of our salvation, through prayer, for success in every battle.[7]

The wording used by the apostle refers to learning how to pray in the Spirit. It is not just a matter of praying about things. It is learning to agree in the spirit with the provision that the Lord makes for us through the Holy Spirit. For instance, if I am praying about healing issues, I don't ask God to heal; I speak out His Word on healing and speak the healing into existence. I take this aggressive approach because God has already made up His mind regarding the healing. Jesus Christ went to the cross to purchase our healing. It is just a matter of agreeing with what the Lord has done. Healing is ours; learning to receive it by faith is our responsibility.

Prayer is a weapon used to stand and fight that which seems unmovable. Endurance is a key element in the process: standing in prayer means taking the focus that is relentless, unshakable, and enduring until the victory. Bible commentator Albert Barnes talks about prayer aided by the Holy Spirit, saying, "No matter how complete the armor; no matter how skilled we may be in the science of war; no matter how courageous we may be, we may be certain that without prayer we shall be defeated. God alone can give the victory; and when the Christian soldier goes forth armed completely for the spiritual conflict, if he looks to God by prayer, he may be sure of a triumph."[8]

To win the battle, we must persist in prayer. Sometimes we are just days, hours, or even minutes from a breakthrough. If you are not seeing results from your prayer time with God, ask Him for wisdom and insight regarding the direction of your prayers. Let your desire be, "Lord, teach me to pray with insight and the intelligence and influence of the Holy Spirit." Stay with it, and don't give up!

Paul used all of these elements of battle to describe the weapons that God has given to us to fight in our spiritual battles. Is it clearer to you now how important the armor is in protecting you and equipping you to fight? When you know how to use these weapons and realize that each piece of the armor complements the others, giving you a complete exterior defense and offense against the enemy, there's no way you can lose!

The Key to Effective Spiritual Warfare

Humans are vessels uniquely structured like God, which is another way we have been given an advantage over our adversaries. We were created for intimate relationship with God and others. The spirit, soul, and body are designed to receive and transfer power, which comes from God. It's His power that enables us to act with strength to defeat the devil and all his forces of darkness. More importantly, it enables us to connect with the Lord (and others) in very deep and meaningful ways. Herein lies the key to effective spiritual warfare: establishing intimacy with God. In God's presence we are safe. My kids love to play outside. I notice that if anything threatens them, even a butterfly, they come running to Daddy. We are the same. We long to know the soothing and comforting voice of our heavenly Father, who takes away the accusatory threats of the enemy.

The human body is designed to know God in a personal way. The life of a believer is built upon what we receive from God via His Spirit to our spirit. This vital connection is like the umbilical chord of a baby. The life of the baby in the womb is dependent on its bond to the mother. In the same way, we are healthy if our union to God remains open and free. This relationship with the Lord is cultivated as we learn to communicate with Him from Spirit to spirit. (See John 4:24 MSG.) We are liberated by His Spirit's presence in our spirit. Can you see how our unique structure helps us defeat our enemy?

We were created by God with natural ability to survive and overcome threats to hurt us. The spirit connects us to the Life Force of the universe, the tongue is a creative force that gives us the power to speak life and death, the heart and soul function as a wellspring of life, the mind manufactures and distributes truth, the eyes are a compass of discernment, the ears are receptors to the Father's voice, the hands are an extension of God's touch, and the body is the residence of God. Let's look at each of these natural abilities individually to get a better picture.

The *tongue* is a vital force because it holds the power of life and death (Proverbs 18:21). With the tongue, we either curse ourselves and others or bless in the same manner. In the same way that God spoke and created the universe, we form our world by the words we speak. (See Gen. 1.) We speak into our lives building blocks of reality every day, and we are either freed or snared by the words of our mouths.

The *heart* is the core, or the will, of a person. Our will is corrupted by sinful nature until our nature is transformed by Christ after we become born again. Yet the will must be trained to yield to God, which it learns to do as we trust God and find Him to be true. At all times the will must be carefully guarded and undergirded with truth, but it is interesting that the more we give over the rights to our lives to the Lord, the more purposeful and fulfilling our lives become.

The *mind* is the center for knowledge. We know what we know because we learn to believe. Combined with the will, the mind must be trained and renewed daily. The mind is created to be filled with knowledge. We expand the mind by sowing righteous thoughts and reaping virtue in our judgments. The battle in the mind is won as we actively focus on the goodness of God.

The *eyes* are the compass for discernment. When we plow a path through in the enemy's territory, discernment is our guide. We see with our physical eyes things in this natural world, but we also "see" with spiritual eyes, which give us spiritual insight or discernment. The eyes are the window of the soul. Vision provides judgment to us for our surroundings and the tactics of the enemy.

The *ears* are the receptors to the voice of God. We hear with the physical ear and the spiritual ear. The physical ear knows the audible voice; the spiritual ear knows the spiritual voice. Jesus said, "My sheep hear My voice . . . and they follow Me" (John 10:27). In other words, His sheep know His voice. Knowing His tone beyond and over the oppressive and deceptive voice of the enemy is the key to sound mental health. The Father's voice is the sound of perfect love, and it edifies the soul; the accuser's voice is the sound of fear, condemning the soul.

The *hands* are the point of touch. The touch of God brings healing and justice. The finger of God (Luke 11:20) reflects His direction and His presence. God uses our hands to do the same. The hands serve as a point of contact through which the virtue of the Lord travels. God is into hugs and embraces!

The *body* is defined as the temple of God in the New Testament scriptures (1 Cor. 3:16). Our bodies are living sacrifices to the Lord. Our service to Him is a form of housekeeping of the body—the way we keep house or take care of the body is a reflection of worship to God.

Both the armor of God, which portrays our image in Him, and the natural resources we are equipped with to fight the enemy are part of the arsenal God has empowered us with to defeat our adversary. We are called to utilize these weapons to tear down strongholds, to build up our faith, and to fill the void in our hearts and minds with truth. All of these resources enable us to overcome the nature and tactics of our enemy.

The Wiles of the Devil

The aggression and oppression of our enemy, Satan, comes because it is his nature to attack. If we sit back and mind our business like "good little Christians," we will become perfect targets. He will zero in on us with the knowledge that we don't believe in evil or the existence of spiritual forces that seek to destroy us. He is like an annoying fly that keeps buzzing over the food on the table. The fly smells the food and attacks because he wants to feed on it. The fly is not going to leave us alone because we politely shoo it away. The only remedy is to swat the fly (or "swap it," as my four-year-old says) with great authority, knowing the splattering of his body will bring us peace. The prince of the air has a similar strategy. He is going to keep annoying us and oppressing us until he is able to bring us harm.

Satan's subtleness is his specialty. The subtle tactics of our adversary are carried out in manipulative and cunning ways to gain points for his team. He gains ground in our lives by appealing to the needs in our soul and our body. When we are ignorant of his ways and our defense against him, the outcome is that he wins and we lose. He knows what trips our triggers; so, at times, he does not have to work very hard in luring us to entertain evil. He simply takes a need in our lives, such as the need for food, and distorts it into an opportunity for us to become god of our lives. Don't take my word for it; look in Genesis 3 at what happened to Eve during her episode with the serpent.

Here is an example of how his subtlety works, using a spirit of fear to oppress us. If we succumb to temptation and believe the voice of fear in our hearts and minds, it can become a seed that produces doubt regarding God's authority in our present circumstances. Two seeds produce more distorted thinking, and so on. Now the object of fear is greater than the presence of the Lord. Ultimately, the devil's goal is to convince us that the object of our fear is a real event in our future. He promotes the lie as if we have no options but to believe it. If we think, speak, and act in agreement with the fear, then it becomes a real event in our life. The thing we were afraid of transpires in living color by our innocent cooperation and participation with evil.

Much to my demise, I was oblivious to this subtle power of darkness. I did not believe that the enemy had access to me because I was a born-again, Spirit-filled Christian. So, in my mind, there was no way that he had the ability to get to me. Maybe he could tempt me, but that was about it. Now it is true that being covered in the blood of Jesus can protect us from the enemy, but the only glitch was that I was not walking in my divine authority—Christ was not in control of my life—therefore, I left myself uncovered. I was being driven by dark beliefs in the pit of my soul, and my life was wrapped around my goal-oriented, driven lifestyle.

The overall plan of the serpent is to influence us to walk away from God and pursue life on our own terms. Some may say that my temptation to sin is simply my unregenerate or unchanged sinful nature. I agree that the unchanged part of me is a landing strip for the enemy's attack. Satan's use of Peter to voice the will of mankind is a good example of how the enemy gets into our thinking (Matthew 16:23). Moments before Christ rebuked the devil at work in Peter, this bold, impulsive fisherman spoke about the most powerful revelation recorded in the Gospels: Jesus is the Messiah (vv. 15–17). Then Peter messed up that opportunity by sticking his foot in his mouth and declaring that Jesus would not need to be crucified. Peter went from speaking a Holy Spirit inspired declaration to speaking on behalf of Satan himself. This is how the enemy plants seeds of corruption in our thinking and leads us to act on them. It proves how important it is for us to weigh in the balance every thought that rises above the supremacy of the knowledge that Jesus is Lord.

Why do we have thoughts that seem to invade our minds from nowhere? The thought of tragedy to my family or the thought of financial ruin is not a pleasant sensation, nor am I the source from which it springs. I do not wake up trying to create destructive patterns in my life. How could the apostle Paul say that a messenger of Satan was sent to place a thorn in his flesh to prevent him from gaining revelation? (See 2 Cor. 12:7.) Was he just making that up? No, the devil works to challenge our thinking and steer us down a path of destruction.

Do you remember the story of Ananias and Sapphira? They were obviously believers because they had sold their property to be a part of the move of God. Yet before they brought the money to Peter, they decided to take out some to keep for themselves. But Peter knew what they had done, and he asked them why they had allowed Satan to fill their hearts with a lie toward the Holy Spirit (Acts 5:1–6). This is a reflection of how the deceiver works in our thinking and influences us to choose his path. Ananias and Sapphira were not possessed demoniacs; they were ordinary people who were taken captive by the lies of the enemy.

A number of strategies are repetitively launched by Satan. His bags of tricks are cyclical and predictable to the discerning believer. He uses various methods to wear us down, hoping to distract us from dependence on God. Everything he does is an effort to separate us from the loving arms of our heavenly Father. The wiles of the devil that I believe are most consequential are his accusations, his attempt to divide us, his attempt to scare us, his attempt to wound us emotionally, and his attempt to win us.

The Bible says in John's Revelation that the accuser stays before the throne day and night, accusing the brethren (v. 12:10). That's his job. He is constantly trying to discredit us and God. He cleverly presents his argument, as a dishonest used car salesman might, hoping to sway us into buying his bad product. The junk that Satan tries to sell us is false beliefs—he wants to get us to drive away in a lemon filled with them because he knows that down the road that piece of junk will fall apart and blow up in our face. When failure sets in, he hopes we will fall prey to his antics and blame God for our hardship. If we do blame God, we will separate ourselves from Him. Division is like a touchdown in hell. Our evil opponent stands up and hollers every time our choices lead to splitting us apart from God, self, or others. He knows that when we are disconnected our power is diminished. Unity is a great force that drives him out and joins people together to advance the goodness of God. Churches constantly split over minor things that blow up into big arguments. Who wins those battles? If I win, then my brother or sister (in Christ) loses—and ultimately Satan wins.

Another trick the enemy uses is terrorism, or the illusion of pending doom. Lucifer (Satan), in his fallen state, is the original terrorist. He is constantly trying to cast a shadow of fear on people. The prophet Ezekiel said that after Lucifer was banished from heaven, he (the devil) would remain a terror and nothing more (Ezek. 28:19). Satan is a little man with "big man syndrome"; he tries to make himself look a lot bigger than he really is. His ultimate goal is for you to destroy yourself as a result of his shadow. He looms over you, taunting you with thoughts of a gloomy future, hoping you will believe his tyrannical, false gospel. If he can get you to bite, then he'll drag you into harm's way. If he cannot scare you, then he will try to wound you.

Satan often attacks us through other people, but he can also come against us directly. If he cannot knock us off our horse, he will try to get someone else to do it. If that doesn't work, he'll employ self-hatred to take a blow at us. If we believe his lies, we can do more damage to ourselves than he ever does.

Finally, if he cannot hurt us, accuse us, scare us, blame us, or divide us, he will try to win us. He has many toys in his toy box to achieve this goal, and he makes them so attractive that we come to believe they are good for us. Somehow we can rationalize that his invitation to death is an opportunity for a better life. James said that sin brings forth death after lust has fully conceived (James 1:15), yet in our ignorance we give in to sin. Our compromise sets in motion the vicious cycle of grasping for the next greatest sensation for the flesh, which is never wholly satisfied by worldly pleasures.

The appetite of the flesh is a bottomless pit. No sooner have we eaten breakfast than we are already thinking about what we might want for lunch. If we become obsessive or addicted to fleshly appetites, the opposite happens. We no longer have our needs met, but our compulsive actions lead to deep emptiness. Our lives become more and more empty, and it takes more and more to satisfy the flesh; ultimately, the end of the cycle is death.

These tactics are some of the ploys of the devil, but there are countless others. I challenge you to remember that his ultimate aim is to steal, kill, and destroy us, as Jesus stated in John 10:10. Having completed his task, the devil roars like a lion after the kill to bring a fearful reminder that others could easily become his prey. He uses fear and deception to try to defeat us, but he is a liar and a counterfeit. Remember, the Bible says that the devil comes "*as* a roaring lion" (1 Peter 5:8 KJV), but Jesus is "*the* lion of the tribe of Judah" (Rev. 5:5). When you know the enemy and his ways, he cannot harm you—and that's good news!

Opening the Door to Freedom

Out of desperation to find freedom from torment and despair, Christians are starting to wonder if all this business about Satan and his demons is really true. For me, the question is no longer can or will the enemy come after me—he already has come after me, and I know he will continue to come after me, attempting to destroy my life. The fact is that believers and unbelievers alike can be pushed around by the devil. Even Christians can receive temptations or attacks from the enemy and his evil, demonic spirits. It starts with a thought. One of his evil spirits seeks a place in our thinking by introducing negative thoughts into our thoughts. Eventually, if the thought goes unchecked and is not cast down or out, it can grow and produce a full-blown stronghold.

My wife and I have both experienced strongholds, and we have seen them take root in the lives of many of our Christian brothers and sisters as well. You may have had a similar experience in your life. I want to show you how to protect yourself against the devil so that he cannot build his strongholds anywhere near you.

We receive thoughts from several sources. We have our own human thoughts about the events in our world. Much of our thinking is instinctive and related to getting our basic needs met. We also receive thoughts from other people to whom we relate. All of these thoughts make up our *human thinking*. Beyond that, *the enemy* places thoughts in our mind to lead us astray from God. Finally, we can receive thoughts from *God*, which bring life and meaning to our lives.

The enemy is trying to push his agenda on us so that his way of thinking becomes ours. If we yield to this process, over time, we can become oppressed with evil thoughts and end up under the authority of seducing spirits (those that deceive or mislead). That kind of mindset will produce doubt and pull us away from faith in God (1 Tim. 4:1).

I find that, at times, even when I am walking in harmony with God, Satan tries to come against me. If I allow him in, then he comes in. The welcome mat is still on the front porch of our "houses" if our sinful core beliefs are still in us. Even when we are full of God's Spirit, the tempter will try to allure us away from godly thinking and living. We subject ourselves to temptation if we lean on our own strength. Remember, the apostle Paul said, "I do the things I don't want to do, and the things I want to do I do not" (Rom. 7:15, my paraphrase). This passage refers to the age-old battle of the flesh when we are struggling to surrender to the authority of God and learning to flee temptation.

Let's return to Peter's struggle with this battle. In Mark 8:27, Jesus asked His disciples, *"Who do men say that I am?"* Their reply indicated that some believed He was John the Baptist while others believed He was one of the prophets. Jesus then made His appeal more specific by inquiring of them, *"Who do you say that I am?"* to which Peter resounded, *"You are the Christ"* (v. 29). If you recall, only moments later, Jesus made reference to something bad happening to Him in the near future and Peter reprimanded Him for it. Yet Christ didn't rebuke Peter; He rebuked Satan, who was using the mouth of Peter (vv. 32–33).

All of this transpired within the course of a common conversation in a few moments of time. Peter was a believer who had previously cast out devils, yet the enemy used Peter's mouth to speak against Christ. The foundational belief of fear had already been planted in Peter's mind, so it was simple for Satan to get Peter to entertain that thought, and then speak it to Jesus. This core belief, which was a stronghold of fear from the enemy, influenced Peter to deny Christ during the crucifixion (Matt. 26:69–75).

People may want to debate this issue of whether or not the devil comes after us, but to me there is no debate left when your life is on the line. I believe that to debate now would be to deny what the power of the Savior did in my life when He rescued me from hell on earth. He delivered me from a spirit of rebellion and self-hatred, which enabled me to receive the love of my heavenly Father in a deeper way than ever before. That's when my body began to visibly heal. My wife's testimony is similar. She had been tormented with depression from childhood, but she has not been tormented since the Lord delivered her of a spirit of self-hatred. No amount of debate on this issue will change our experience; the matter is a done deal for us. Now our mission is to share God's delivering power with every oppressed person we can get to.

I now know that I have absolute authority over Satan because Christ defeated and disarmed him two thousand years ago on the cross, and He eventually will destroy him (Rev. 20:1–3). So the enemy no longer has authority over me unless I grant it to him; I win by believing in Christ's complete and finished work. You can win, too. Believing Jesus has already won the victory on your behalf will open the prison door for you, just as it did for me.

You Can Have a Quality Life

Learning to discern the difference between good and evil preserves life and could affect an entire generation. When I looked back at my father's side of the family, I realized that they were not Christians; they were heathens. I'm sure that many of my father's struggles could have been avoided, had someone taught him about Jesus. Solomon's message to us in Proverbs is that wisdom, the application of truth, is the key to a quality life. Transformation and discernment are complimentary.

We've talked much about discernment in this book because it is an important part of a transformed life. Something else you should know about discernment is that it comes with pure thinking. Clarity in our understanding comes as we mature in our walk with the Lord. Maturity should never be replaced with a gift or a talent. It is also crucial to remember that warfare against the adversary only works if we are walking in obedience to Christ. If we are violating His Word, then it will not work. God will not bless disobedience to His natural or spiritual laws.

We are putting ourselves at risk if we ignorantly believe we are living for Christ but are in fact disobeying His precepts and commands. The sons of Sceva discovered this truth when they used the name of our Lord flippantly, trying to cast out devils. The men had no power over the enemy because they were not walking in obedience to God. So when they tried to command a demon to come out of a man in Jesus' name, here's what happened:

> *"Answering, the evil spirit said, Jesus I know, and I comprehend Paul, but who are you? And the man in whom the evil spirit resided leaped on them, and overcoming them he was strong against them, so that they fled out of the house naked and wounded."*
> ACTS 19:13–16

Now, I'm not trying to put fear in you. I want you to understand how the devil works to try to get you away from God. If he succeeds because you ignore him or are ignorant of his tricks and strategies, he can gain entrance into your life. So first of all, don't be afraid of this message; the Bible says that God has not given us a spirit of fear, but of power, love, and a sound mind (2 Tim. 1:7). Paul is saying here that you have the same power that raised Jesus from the dead living inside you (Rom. 8:11), you have the love of God in you (1 John 2:5), and you have the mind of Christ. (1 Cor. 2:16.) What a combination to get you out from under the influencing power of the enemy!

If you think that you have some kind of demonic influence coming against you, here are three questions you can ask yourself: (1) Have I tried everything I know of and have access to, from ministry to medicine, to overcome this struggle in my life, but still cannot get free of it? (2) Do I sometimes feel as though someone or something comes over me, or takes me over, to such a degree that I am unable to control my own behavior? (3) Is the way I behave during these episodes radically and completely contradictory to how I would normally choose to behave? If you feel the answer is yes to these questions, then you may want to consider taking some basic steps to get further help.

If you have already been trying to pray for freedom on your own without success, I encourage you to pray for God to lead you to a safe place. Because there is a current movement of people seeking the power of God through the supernatural works of the early church (as seen through the life of Paul), there are many more ministries available to people in need of this type of ministry than there were several years ago. So seek God about where and whom to turn to for help. He will lead you. I suggest that you also speak with your pastor about your situation. If you still need help, we have contacts around the country to network with; maybe we can help you. That is what our ministry is all about, helping others get real and get free. So if you would like to contact our ministry, we will try to assist in guiding you through the process. (Please see our ministry contact information at the end of this book.)

Keep in mind that deliverance is a simple process that involves releasing the oppression of the enemy. We see in the Word that Christ gave all believers authority over evil spirits (Luke 10:19). We simply do what He did. We gather in His name and ask for protection and discernment, we expect the power of the Holy Spirit to guide and direct the process, and whenever we come against evil, we do everything in the name of Jesus as He instructed His disciples to do in the Gospels. This approach to ministry is not complicated, just very direct. Remember, Christ's atonement lays the foundation for deliverance, opens the door for cleansing, and offers us the power to exchange the enemy's oppression with freedom.

During ministry we also walk through each area of a person's life and help them release the oppression. The process takes different courses of direction, depending on the person's needs, but before we get into that process, we ask the person who is subject to evil to repent for allowing the presence to control them. When they repent, we come against the force of darkness until it is removed.

The forgiveness issue creates confusion for some because sometimes people do not understand why we expect them to repent before deliverance. Asking for forgiveness for entertaining evil on whatever level we have chosen is about taking personal responsibility for our wrongs. Even though we may be oblivious to our sin, it is still our liability before God. John said that if we confess our sin, then God is faithful to forgive it (1 John 1:9). Our confession becomes a building block for personal freedom; God is then compelled to meet us in our struggle. True change of heart, which is the foundation for biblical repentance, begins with our admission of sin or wrongdoing.

After the deliverance experience, repentance should continue. Repentance and change do not end with confession or admittance of guilt. We cannot just say we are sorry one minute and expect everything to be better the next. Often there are very real consequences we must face as a result of our actions, and in some cases, those consequences bring long-term effects. For instance, if a woman has bitterness because her best friend betrayed her, she first needs to repent to the Lord for hanging onto the offense and then repent to the woman with whom she is offended. Over time, she will have to work out any natural consequences that stemmed from her actions.

If we have created breeches in relationships, we must seek those people out and try to repair the damage. If we are holding grudges against others who hurt us, then we must let go of those issues of bitterness and release all parties for hurting us. All of these actions reflect true repentance.

Repentance is a deep work. It is an ever increasing unfolding of the layers of a person's heart, which involves exchanging the darkness for God's light. He shines the light on us, illuminating our obvious struggle with sin so that we can get in line with His established order, and then He invites us to change. If we lay down our weakness before Him, He replenishes us with real strength. The sanctification process does take time and dedication, but the ideal plan from here is that we become new—the old passes away and our heart changes.

Learning to repent arms us to fight the spiritual battle we must face in order to be healed, restored, and made new. Renewal is a process, but the more we apply the principle of repentance and exercise forgiveness, the more open and cleansed our spirits will become before God. Each step we take is an act of faith, but God will meet us every step of the way, empowering us to yield to Him and disarm the enemy.

Something very important to remember is that, after deliverance, we will have holes, or gaps, left in our soul that we need to fill up with the Word of God. We do not want to be at risk for more evil to fill those gaps again, so we must renew our minds by meditating on God's Word. (See Matt. 12:43–45.) When we fill our minds with scripture, that Word inside us strengthens us, enabling us to defeat the enemy again during future attacks. Jesus Himself overcame the attacks of the adversary with the weapon of God's Word.

Deliverance was initially meant to be a ministry of love from a compassionate Savior who desires to rescue His people. We see in the Bible that Jesus' approach was forceful toward evil spirits but gentle toward those being delivered. His example should be our model. If you have ever been subject to hostility in deliverance ministry, it was done in error. The end result should always be your freedom and God's glory.

Prayer:

Father God, I run to You! I seek Your heart for the freedom of my soul. Only You can set me free. I have been taken captive. I recognize the enemy's advance in my life, and I repent. I no longer want any part or collaboration with evil. I want all evil out of my life. I ask You to search my heart. Show me if I have allowed the enemy to build strongholds in my life, and if so, where. Reveal to me the roots of my sin. Open my heart and clear away any blinders.

I ask You to forgive me for rationalizing the evil in my life, for making it seem okay. Deliver me, Lord. Bring me out of darkness and into the light. You are the only One who can empower me to be free. I ask in the name of Jesus Christ that the power of darkness be broken in my life. Free me from the clutches of evil. Release me from the enemy's grip.

Thank You for Jesus, who overcame the devil and gave us authority to do the same. I stand before You today as a blood-bought son/daughter of the King of kings, and I rise to take my position in Christ. You are my Savior and Lord. I shall serve no other gods. You alone shall be Captain of my soul. You are the Commander in Chief, and I stand ready to follow Your orders. Lead me into battle to crush the enemy. Praise God who reigns above all! I am victorious over death, hell, and destruction because our Lord is not dead but rose from death to be seated in heavenly places on the throne at the right hand of our Father. I count it all joy to serve You! Amen.

CHAPTER 7

GET OUT OF THE JUNGLE OF DESTRUCTION

Breaking Generational Patterns

Say it isn't so. The landscape is the same, the people are the same, the experience is familiar, and the outcome is definitely the same. I lose no matter how hard I try to win. Yep, I have seen this trail and been down this road before. It feels like I am going around the same mountain, over and over. I look out the window and everything is too familiar. I recognize this setup as if I stepped onto a Universal Studios Hollywood set. I keep seeing the same up and down patterns in my life; they are too much to handle. What is happening?

AFTER A FAILED BUSINESS THAT TURNED INTO BANKRUPTCY, relationships that produced more pain than strength, ministry experiences that produced heartache and confusion, a declining marriage, thinking more about death than life, and a diseased body that I could not get healed, I finally got the picture.

I was following the footsteps of my earthly father much more than my heavenly Father. I knew along the way that things were supposed to be different, but I never seemed able to break free. I was reliving the life of my forefathers as if their bad luck and hard times were my destiny.

I was shocked to discover that I was living as though I was under a generational curse. Because I thought my salvation experience with Christ had ransomed me from such misery, it was very difficult for me to fathom that my problems were connected to the failures, frustrations, and sins of my forefathers. The notion of generational curses gave me thoughts of Ouija boards forecasting doom and warlocks casting spells on people from dark, damp dungeons—but my attitude about the matter did not change my reality. I was walking in the dark and thought I was in the light. I could not understand why every time I was sure I was going to make an advance in my life, I would hit a brick wall. This pattern of unending frustrations led to my discovery of the generational effect of curses. The pattern made a lot of sense when I examined it. The truth was that I was repeating the very same self-destructive patterns in my life that my father and other extended family members had lived under for years. I was reaping the consequences of the cursed living of my forefathers, not the blessings of my Savior, Jesus Christ.

It was a reality check for me to awaken to the fact that my life was not full of the blessings of God. It was an even deeper revelation to realize that my rebellion, my stiffness toward Him, had opened the door for this to happen. God is merciful to allow us to experience the fruit of our decisions. He teaches us with natural consequences, hoping to get our attention so that He can introduce us to a greater reality—His grace.

Discovering that I had made a mess of things and that this pattern had been in my family line for generations was an act of God's mercy. It was like learning that I lived on a farm where contaminated water caused health problems. God did not contaminate the water; the actions of people caused the water to be polluted. God provides pure water, but our actions make it dirty. God is merciful, looking for a way to make provision in our lives. God handled my generational problems similarly by revealing to me the destructive patterns in the way my forefathers lived and offering me an opportunity to be free.

The real point is that Jesus Christ overcame the curse, "having become what we were, in our behalf, 'a curse' [because of our sinful nature], that we might cease to be a curse. Not merely accursed (in the concrete), but a curse in the abstract, bearing . . . the whole sin of our race.[1]

Jesus' advancement makes a way for us to overcome all of the curses (or sins) that our forefathers produced. But progress beyond those patterns must be appropriated by our faith. We cannot live in the land of freedom and promise until we get up and walk through the gate of faith. We must learn to appropriate the goodness of God. He does not just plop it in our lap. He requires that we join Him and walk with Him in agreement with His provision.

What I find is that my stinking thinking and unlearned ways prevent me from entering into the promised land of milk and honey. Deep down in my heart I know that I belong in a better place, but breaking free from the things I learned as a kid takes some effort.

Ungodly generational thinking prevents us from entering into our spiritual inheritance and authority as followers of Christ. You may say, "But I am redeemed from the curse by the sacrifice of Christ." Yes, I agree with that, but let me ask you a question. Why are we still repeating and perpetuating the sins of our forefathers? We fall short of breaking free from their patterns because we are never awakened to the greater reality—the grace of God that is available to save and deliver us from a life of destruction. I came into this revelation because of my failure to prevent and end destructive patterns in my own life. The same sins of rebellion, addiction, anger, impatience, infirmity, and sexual dysfunction from my family line also showed up in my adult life. I became enslaved to the same junk my dad was a slave to, even after my radical, born-again experience. What was up with that? How could this be?

Not me! This was my youthful claim before marriage and children. I did not want to repeat the same patterns of my father. I truly and deeply desired health, wholeness, and to live a life of righteousness. So I became a born-again Christian, applied myself to the study of God's Word, was filled with His Spirit, spoke in tongues (1 Cor. 14:5; Jude 1:20) as a young man, attended a charismatic Christian university, earned a master's degree in marriage counseling, went to the right church, married the right girl, and hung out with the right people. To my knowledge, I was living the life of faith and righteousness that I was supposed to.

What was missing? I truly believe the understanding I was missing was a deep revelation of the power of the abiding presence of the Holy Spirit. Throughout my Christian life, I was taught a form of religion without the power of God, and I was not taught how to break free from the past. Modern psychology has been a catalyst in bringing people to the awareness of the need to overcome the past, but I do not believe that modern psychology is the answer. It is rooted in humanism, which causes people to spiral into an abyss of being absorbed in self, becoming all that "I" can be, while in complete charge of their life. This is the opposite of God's plan for us, which is total dependence on Him.

What we need is transformation of character, not self-actualization. That's the problem with humanism. It attempts to bring awareness and meaning apart from confronting the rebellious nature of man and the evil presence of Satan. Man must be brought into the light (God). Darkness (Satan) must be consumed by the light, not shrouded with the "shadow of enlightenment." Man's only hope is to encounter the real living God. He is the only One who can save us. Self-awareness is a bottomless pit that creates an unending search for answers that do not exist within the heart of self. We don't have the answers; Jesus does. The Incarnate Son of God is the One who delivers us from our reality. He is the truth, and it is truth that frees us, not a microscopic vision of self. We need to release these generational patterns, and the only way to do so is to become somebody new, discovering our God-potential not our human potential.

We were created for greatness. The journey to greatness comes as we recognize that our Creator set up this world in a special order. If we violate God's order, then we produce problems for ourselves and must face the consequences of our actions. On the other hand, if we walk in God's plan, He will restore us. We cannot fix ourselves. God alone has the power to raise us up to supernatural potential. We see evidence of His restorative power in the Old Testament. It is the story of God's steadfast devotion to an unknown, undeserving people who rose to greatness because of the provision from God—through many generations, He delivered them from self-destruction. God takes pleasure in raising the weakest of the weak to a place of prominence in His kingdom.

Here is the dilemma: We know of the blessings, we have tasted them, and we believe they exist; but our lives resemble the product of ruin rather than renewal. We passionately desire a better life, but we can't find our way out of this jungle of destruction. We live in the age of prosperity, but inside we know something is wrong. Perhaps we have never considered that we could be living under a curse—after all, we do see a measure of external success in our lives. (If we tend to evaluate our lives in this way, we should remember, the rich young ruler did not enter God's kingdom because he was consumed with his material possessions; see Matt. 19:16–22.) Yet the question we must honestly ask ourselves is, do we see the life of God being reproduced in us?

Jesus told his disciples to pray that the kingdom of God would come on the earth. Jesus also said the kingdom of God is within us. So bringing God's kingdom to earth is about reproducing the life of God within believers. Our goal is to experience an active, nonstop reproduction of God's grace in our lives so that we walk daily in the blessings of God. Though some Christians may spend their days marching around the mountain in tears, taking tours on the wilderness trail, God's desire is that we walk on the road of salvation, not devastation.

Generational curses don't just happen; they come from our repeated rebellion toward God. We saw earlier that a curse is the consequence of sin resulting from God's judgment (or separation from God). In other words, when we violate His standard, we bring judgment upon ourselves. God's judgment differs from His discipline (Heb. 12:6–7), because discipline serves more as a warning, while judgment yields a life pattern of failures and frustrations that constitute a lack of God's favor. God uses both His judgment and His discipline to save our lives. Let me give you an example of what I mean.

If we have a child who constantly wants to play in the street, we take measures to protect him. First we may warn him that if he goes into the street again, he will receive a consequence such as having to sit in time out. If he continues, the punishment may become harsher, like a spanking or being grounded from playing outside. If he still continues, the discipline may become more stringent. But God forbid that he goes into the street and an accident occurs. The day his violation of our standard causes his destruction, he is under our judgment; but that is not what we desired for him. We wanted him to live a full life in the context of our safety. The other side of this example is that if he heeds our correction, he lives a long life with our approval, favor, and blessing.

Before we go on, let me clarify something. I do not believe we come under a curse if we commit a one-time sin. Christ gave His life so that we could overcome our sin. If we deal with the sin by repenting before God and seeking His forgiveness, then a stronghold does not develop. The concern here is patterns of sin, not single issues of sin. In addition, I am not referring to those people who are being persecuted for the cause of Christ. Their persecution is not a curse; it is a blessing—not because it is pleasant, but because it produces the opportunity for God's glory to manifest. When I speak of generational curses, I am speaking of those self-imposed struggles from which we cannot break free.

Because we faced such deep issues in our lives, my wife and I waded through various counseling programs, searching for answers. What we discovered was, numerous generational roads led to our present problems; the issues our parents and their parents had dealt with were the same things we were wrestling. Fear, anger, rejection, jealousy, bitterness, addiction, and poverty were the strongholds our ancestors had battled, and those curses were showing up in our lives as well, despite all the measures we had taken to prevent them.

Much of the work we had done through counseling and related programs paved a way for us to break these generational curses. I discovered that my lifestyle had robbed me of the blessings and birthright promised to me in Christ. The idea of counseling sounded simple and easy enough, so we decided to find out what the generation before us had done wrong and then change our lives for the better. But it didn't quite work out that way.

Every time we pressed in to learn more, we hit roadblocks. At first we thought if we were more aware of the generational sins, we would be able to overcome them; but awareness actually caused us to spiral downward at times. Then we thought if we gained further insight into what caused them, we could conquer them. That didn't seem to help either. Eventually we realized that neither awareness nor understanding were enough. So we went back to the starting point. (Just because you know that chocolate is a weakness does not mean you can resist it. You need power to overcome it.) In the long run, our breakthroughs came because we encountered the supernatural power of God. He reached inside us and touched us, causing a shift in our lives and an empowerment to overcome. Otherwise, we would still be stuck.

The goal of this chapter is to lay a foundation for dealing with the generational sins of our forefathers. We are not bashing our fathers, mothers, or grandparents for their sin. Our objective is to divorce ourselves from sin, not people. We are not laying blame at the feet of those who have passed away, either. We are taking responsibility for the sin produced before us, laying it at the foot of the cross with the expectation that God will empower us and those who follow after us to live in righteousness.

Submit, Release, and Receive

Jehovah passed by before him and proclaimed, Jehovah! Jehovah God, merciful and gracious, long-suffering, and abundant in

goodness and truth, keeping mercy for thousands, forgiving iniq-
uity and transgression and sin, and who will by no means clear the
guilty, visiting the iniquity of fathers on the sons, and on the sons
of sons, to the third and to the fourth generation.

EXODUS 34:6, 7

At first glance, this scripture paints a bleak picture. It seems to be
saying that sin is a powerful force that creates an unstoppable pattern
of destruction. How can that be good? How is that a reflection of
longsuffering and mercy?

God is not double-minded. Sin threatened to destroy the human
race, but it did not happen. The course of our demise was altered by
the goodness of One—the Creator. God could have turned us over
to the consequences of our sin, but did not. Instead, He unfolded
His plan of redemption. Throughout history, He has demonstrated
His genuine commitment to emancipating us from slavery to sin. Yet
at the same time, God knows that if we go unchecked in our sin, we
can destroy ourselves.

It is hard for those of us who came from dysfunctional families to
think of God as fair, that Father God governs the world with justice
balanced with mercy, unlike the events in our childhood homes. Our
distorted perception of justice is overlaid with cruelty and hatred
because of the sin of our fathers. Many times our own hurt prevents
us from seeing the goodness of God in His justice.

God set us up for freedom from the consequences of our sin and
the sins of our fathers. He does this by governing the world according
to His spiritual and natural laws. God's law is there for our protection, not to dominate us. He wants us to be free to choose His ways.
On the other hand, sin entered by the deception of Satan and the
rebellion of man.

Sin, the presence of darkness, leads to death and must be washed
out of our lives. God's law magnifies our sin and our sinful condition.
The process of washing out sin and the consequences of sin comes
as we realize our need for Him to cleanse us. His law as written in
the Old Testament, or Old Covenant, provides the foundation for

the conditions of His relationship with us. That law cannot rescue us from our dilemma but points to our need to be utterly dependent on God.

God's requirements come with provisions. In other words, the expectations of God come with directions for the fulfillment of His laws (His principles or judgments). But God is not a taskmaster. He is interested in our welfare, and He set the law in place to protect us from destruction and failure. Can you imagine traveling on a winding mountain road late at night without warning signs? That would spell sure disaster. Just as speed limits protect us from endangerment, so God's law sets in motion eternal standards that exist for our security.

God took the lead by assuming responsibility for our redemption. Solomon said the best thing we can do is get wisdom about how God operates. (See Prov. 4:5, 7; 16:16.) Solomon realized the value of God's good judgments. Contained within each principle is destiny to fulfill it, if we choose to learn.

The sacrificial system that God used to implement His law provided a means to correcting the problem of sin in the hearts of men. Ultimately, the medium of sacrifice empowers us to change and walk according to God's law. His goal was to give us both the blessing of His wisdom and the power to implement it. We play an entirely different game if we know we are going to win.

The mercy of God came in His faithfulness to the covenant He established with man, covenant being an agreement between two parties. He agreed to provide our redemption if we would obey His laws. This contract produced the foundation of our relationship with God. Throughout the ages God has been faithful to fulfill His part of the arrangement. It's mankind who has failed miserably to keep their part. We all fall short. Thank God for giving us grace through Jesus Christ! The climax of this plan came as the Messiah, Jesus Christ, was born into the world as the final sacrifice for our sins. The atoning death of Jesus made a perfect way for us to be pardoned and live as free men and women. The deal is done and we are free—if and only if. The if is important because we must respond to the conditions of

God. We cannot save ourselves, but we must grab the lifeline if we want to experience salvation.

Rebellion hinders God's plan. The era of grace established by the Son of God has promoted the opportunity for our freedom. We stand emancipated, unless we continue to choose slavery. American history records that, even after legally being freed, many slaves were too afraid to seek out their freedom once the Civil War ended. Their whole generation was standing at the threshold of a brand-new life. They had no vision of what was ahead, and some actually chose to remain under the bondage of the past. That is hard to believe, but we are no different if we continue to live by the destructive patterns of past generations and remain slaves to the taskmaster, Satan, when our Savior has pardoned and freed us.

> *Do not yield your members as instruments of unrighteousness to sin, but yield yourselves to God, as one alive from the dead, and your members as instruments of righteousness to God. For sin shall not have dominion over you, for you are not under Law, but under grace. What then? Shall we sin because we are not under Law, but under grace? Let it not be!*
>
> ROMANS 6:13–15

God wants us to be directed by a greater force than the power of sin. He wants us to become empowered by His love. That is why Jesus came to earth. He is interested in eradicating the power of sin and the consequences of it. He takes no pleasure in our being under the curses of past generations. He wants us to live free from them. This passage tells us how—by yielding. God's hope is that we willingly submit to Him, release the past, and receive His mercy.

Uprooting Generational Patterns

Like it or not, we are a product of Maw and Paw from past generations. Each succeeding generation makes a contribution to the lifestyle and the purposes for life, and that contribution includes their sins. The iniquity of our forefathers (their sin) is replicated by each generation until there is a reason for change. The product of sinful generations eventually produces sin patterns that are destructive, and families often keep these patterns going unless they find some reason to do otherwise. The fact is that people do not change unless they encounter a reason to alter their path. God gives them the best reason—He interrupts this destructive path with the gospel, the Good News.

The "God news" is that we don't have to follow the party line and destroy ourselves like the generations before us. The presence of iniquity is only overcome by grace, which empowers us to be transformed; otherwise, we follow the rest of the herd to slaughter. The power of the good news is that God can and does take a godless generation and transform it into one filled with righteousness and supernatural authority from on high. This process is a deliberate plot of the Lord. He works all things out for our good if we pay attention to His lead.

Keep in mind that I am speaking to those who inherited dysfunction, not those who came from blessing. Anyone who was fortunate to receive a God-filled heritage is truly blessed. This is a blessing that is built on a strong foundation. That foundation sets the stage for the blessed to inhabit the earth and share the wealth of the blessing with those who were less fortunate. This is a good thing, yet even the blessed often need to uproot generational patterns and clean out storage sheds and the cellars of life. It is a good practice to cleanse the house before we move into it, regardless of the inherited condition.

As recorded in the Gospels, Jesus explained the kingdom of God through many parables. The most prominent parable, which unlocks the key to understanding all other parables, is the parable of the sower, the seed, and the soil. The story centers on a Sower (God) who sows His seed (the Word) into the soil (the people of God). For various reasons the seed does or does not grow, and does or does not bear fruit (Matt. 13:3–8, 18–23). This story gives the reason we do or do not inherit blessings from our generations before us.

If they were God-filled generations, they were a people who were good soil and accepted the Word of God and prospered for it. But if they were bad soil, meaning hard, shallow, full of weeds and thorns, then the Word of God was not accepted or it got choked out by the weeds in the garden of their heart. This type of soil became fallow ground and the Word of God did not grow, so there was no production of life. The fruit of this soil was thorns, hardness, dryness, tares (false grain), and weeds. (See Matt. 13:24–30 KJV.) This pattern will continue until Someone uproots the bad seed and breaks up the fallow ground.

Bad soil produces a barren field. Bad growth creates unhealthy and lifeless crops. Physically, people starve and go hungry because of the lack of good water and good food. This lifeless cycle is a curse that comes because the soil did not receive, not because the sower did not sow. Eventually, those bad seeds become rooted and grow into something fruitless unless the seed is removed and another is planted in its place. This is true spiritually as well.

Generational curses in our lives do not just show up one day. They are produced because we do not allow the soil of our heart to be broken and prepared for receiving the seed, the Word of God. We resist the Word and come into agreement with the iniquity of our fathers. This produces a curse, and our land becomes unfruitful because of it. The good news is that there's a way to break up the barren land and receive the blessing of plenty. Before we look at it, I want to emphasize that unfruitfulness in our lives doesn't just happen.

> *As the bird by wandering, as the swallow by flying, so the curse without cause shall not come.*
>
> PROVERBS 26:2

See, there is a reason for the failures and dark history. The droppings of evil do not just land on our head as the bird flies over us. The generations before us engaged in evil, which brought separation from God. Here are a number of clearly marked sin-patterns recorded in the Bible that produce consequences for God's people.

Idolatry: Seeking and Trusting Other Gods

Paul said in Romans 1:25, "They changed the truth of God into a lie, and they worshiped and served the created thing more than the Creator, who is blessed forever." Idolatry leads us to trust others and the things of this world more than God. We are fragile creatures. We seek to find security and oftentimes get into trouble, trying to meet a genuine need. Our actions may seem innocent, but let's look at them a bit further.

If squeezed by life's circumstances, whom do we turn to? Who becomes our "savior" when times get tough? When we deal with life issues, the actions we take indicate whom we really trust. I made my life an open book when it came to my issues. I turned to anybody who would give me answers when I was crippled with illness and broken down emotionally. In so doing, I acted the same way most of the church would—it is not that we do not seek God but that we often seek Him last.

Idolatry involves trust and allegiance. To whom are we loyal? Whom are we following and who gets our devotion? God is passionate for one thing—our hearts. He wants our whole lives to be centered on and wrapped up in Him, not relegated to spending just a few quiet minutes a week with Him. We cry, "Just give me Jesus," and He cries, "Just give Me your heart."

We are walking in idolatry when someone or something else in our lives receives more of our devotion than God does. I have heard Christians respond to this viewpoint by saying, "But I attend church every time the doors are open, and give my tithe to foreign missions." They are offended when you question the motivation behind their acts of service. While good works are important, we cannot base our devotion to God on our works of service or the level of our social status. You can be a good person and never be devoted to God. Devotion comes from passion, and passion comes from relationship.

Passion is that uncontrollable desire we have to pursue. No, I'm not talking about the urge you get at two o'clock in the morning when you stumble into the kitchen looking for milk and cookies.

I am referring to the longing in your soul. What do you cry out for? Do you have any fire in your belly? What consumes you when you daydream at work and during the pastor's eloquent message on Sunday morning? If your church life were taken away tomorrow, what would be left? Your answer to these questions indicates what is driving your relationship with God. If there is no passion in your relationship with Him, then what you have is not a God-centered devotion to the Almighty Creator of the world, but a moral obligation to someone who may or may not be irreplaceable in your life.

What does this have to do with generational curses? If the generations before us were idolatrous, idolatry will show up in our lives. For instance, on my father's side of the family, there were only a few believers. Most others were rebellious toward God, and as a result, they struggled with alcoholism, adultery, and a host of other problems. Like clockwork, the same problems showed up in my life and my siblings' lives. We were taught that you overcome life's challenges with hard work, so we dedicated ourselves to our work, expecting to fulfill our dreams. However, as I discovered, it takes much more than hard work to fulfill those dreams. God's intervention is our only hope. In my case, my family was exposed to the goodness of God, but not all of us received it.

Sometimes generations dedicate themselves to things like hard work, education, creativity, religion, or forms of humanism. Entire cultures wrap around these institutions, and history repeats itself. Each generation is given an opportunity to find its God-filled destiny, but not all choose it. It is up to the present generation to choose. The question is to whom will we devote ourselves?

God is devoted to us because He is the promise keeper. He is the One who chooses to follow after us. He will not fail us, and He never gets tired of extending His mercy to us. But we must get real and recognize these patterns and tear down everything that stands in the way of our devotion to Him. *Tear down the idols and replace them with passion for God and God alone*—that is my cry.

Occultism: Seeking after Knowledge and Enlightenment apart from the Work of the Cross

Now the works of the flesh are clearly revealed, which are: adultery, fornication, uncleanness, lustfulness, idolatry, sorcery, hatreds, fightings, jealousies, angers, rivalries, divisions, heresies, envyings, murders, drunkennesses, revelings, and things like these; of which I tell you before, as I also said before, that they who do such things shall not inherit the kingdom of God.

GALATIANS 5:19–21

The cousin to idolatry is occultism, or sorcery, as Paul indicates in the passage above. Occultism is a controversial subject in today's society because there is an ongoing argument over the very definition of the occult and whether its practices are truly evil.

As Christians, we must recognize the word *occult* is associated with witchcraft. In biblical times, practicing witchcraft involved consulting mediums in seeking answers for problems. The mediums were used to control or manipulate circumstances. Times have not changed. People continue seeking mediums to control and manipulate circumstances in their lives. The argument surrounding occultism opens the door to other questionable behavior as well.

Some believe that all doctors and the practice of any medicine or psychology are associated with the occult. Others believe, if the practice helps people alleviate suffering, it is okay. Still others label everything not defined by science as New Age. I would agree that there are many practices that leave individuals confused and frustrated, but I believe the Bible gives us the best approach.

In the book of Acts, Paul went to Ephesus on a missionary journey, but his ministry to this city included a major upheaval over idolatry and sorcery. Wealthy silversmiths who made money from the production of idols began losing money after Paul arrived because the people were turning away from their practices and turning to God. Their change of heart, along with the silversmiths' loss of revenue, created a commotion in the town (Acts 19:26–30).

Later on, Paul gave the people some advice about the issue. He said, "For you were once darkness, but now you are light in the Lord; walk as children of light" (Eph. 5:8). Paul's admonition persuades me that anything I get involved in—medical care, personal improvement, entertainment, religious practices, or relationships—should be done in God's light. If the practice or ritual is not done in God's light, then the source needs to be considered. I personally trust God for everything but do not direct Him on how He makes provisions. Of course, I am not making a blanket statement about doctors or any other health care practitioners. I am only asserting that it is our responsibility to hear from God what route we are to take when seeking medical help. Seek God first in every situation, and He will show you what to do.

If my forefathers had been involved in occultist activities, then it would be up to me to end the cycle by abandoning every possible form of sorcery. Whatever my ancestors' tendency was in this arena, I must be on guard against and stay totally away from. They may have been involved in certain organizations that do not believe in God or cultural rituals that do not glorify God, or they could have sought enlightenment from spirit guides (another ungodly practice). Whatever the case, my life needs to reflect complete submission to the only Lord and true God, Jesus Christ. The only way to break free from the consequences of an occultist sin pattern is to abandon all forms of allegiance to alternative sources of power.

Rebellion: The Unwillingness to Submit to God

> *Fools are afflicted because of their rebellion, and because of their iniquities.*
>
> PSALM 107:17

Rebellion includes all forms of lawlessness, as well as general irreverence toward God and authority. We often deify the rebel because he or she tears down tyranny and rides on high without accountability. But the truth is, the rebel participates in lawlessness and destroys the moral fabric of our society. The rebel is responsible for breaking up families, creating crime, and destroying the innocence of the world. Unless those in rebellion are stopped, they will continue to take advantage of the weak and adversely affect society.

Rebellion is dangerous because it is progressive. If my father's sin goes unchecked, then I pick up where he left off and eventually my son will add to the problem by continuing to walk in rebellion. The further we separate from God's laws and ways, the more destructive and lawless we become. We see this pattern during the reign of many of the Old Testament kings. If the king was from an ungodly heritage, his leadership produced increasing lawlessness until finally God had to send a messenger to bring truth back into the picture.

Christ approached the rebel with strength. He took Peter, who was a local rebel of his time, and spoke into his life. Jesus did not quarantine Peter; He reached into Peter's heart and called him out of rebellion and into a place of submission. Jesus used the unbridled strength of Peter to break him. Then He filled Peter with His own strength, remaking him into a man who became a pillar for the early church.

God has a special place in His heart for the rebels of society, but just as Peter had to learn to submit, so must they all.

Perversion/Immorality: Seeking Gratification above Perfect Love

For this cause, God gave them up to dishonorable affections.
ROMANS 1:26

Paul went on in Romans 1 to list the behaviors that follow the sins of perversion. We have a tendency to red-flag certain sins as more sinful than others. For example, we may consider sexual sin to be more sinful than an excessive appetite for food. But to God it is all the same—sin. So I am not going to list here the sins Paul described; you can read about them for yourself in that chapter. But know this: if we are struggling with sexual sin or with gluttony or with any other kind of perverted or immoral sin, it is because we do not know perfect love. Nothing can satisfy us like the perfect love of God.

Each layer of perverted, immoral behavior our forefathers partici-
pated in creates obstacles for us to sort through. To participate in a
perversion is to turn an appropriate behavior into an offensive one.
We use things like sex, eating, drinking alcohol, and even working
as a means to gain pleasure and satisfaction. If our actions lead to
indulgence or we take things to extremes, that which was acceptable
becomes twisted. The marker for sin is not what our personal comfort
level is, but what the original design for the activity was according
to its Creator. For instance, sex was not created for the purpose the
world presents to us. Sex was fashioned by God to be an enjoyment
and a blessing to husbands and wives, enabling them to become one
by being connected emotionally and physically in a loving marriage
relationship. The world has perverted this concept.

Generational perversion builds with each new level of compromise.
The illicit activity in which our forefathers engaged in "the good old
days" is considered simple nonsense compared to what is broadcast
into the homes of most Americans today. Violence, hatred, adultery,
incest, homosexuality, gossip, and all other forms of dysfunction are
presented as normal behaviors on the everyday primetime television
shows. Society is now saturated with these behaviors because we have
not turned away from our fathers' sins. Instead, we have amplified
them. For this reason many people are hurt, abused, and oppressed
in their families.

Words: The Power of Life and Death

> By [the tongue] we bless God, even the Father. And by [the tongue]
> we curse men, who have come into being according to the image
> of God. Out of the same mouth proceeds blessing and cursing. My
> brothers, these things ought not to be so.
>
> JAMES 3:9, 10

We are often flippant with our words. We say what we don't mean
and mean what we don't say. We need help big-time in this area. Our
words are the expression of our beliefs. Say something often enough

and it becomes believable. Take, for instance, the words spoken over us as children. Perhaps you were told, "You will never amount to anything" or "You get on my nerves" or "Stop crying before I give you something to cry about" or the old adage "Children should be seen and not heard." Statements such as these can be deeply humiliating and wounding. Interestingly, the same words spoken over us as children, we often repeat to our own children, even though we swore we would never utter them to our kids.

When harsh, demeaning words are spoken over us, they hinder us from developing self-esteem and confidence and can cause us to form an inaccurate self-perception; on the other hand, when encouraging, affirmative words are spoken over our lives, they serve as building blocks of inner strength and confidence, eventually yielding a deep sense of value and self-worth. I don't know how many ministry sessions I have had with people to help them break loose from the words spoken over them as children. Sometimes those words carry more than emotional problems; they act as a self-fulfilling prophecy.

Reversing the damage of words comes as we hear the healing words of God in our own heart. His Word replaces the garbage spoken over us and empowers us to speak the truth in love to others

Passing the Torch

The Bible clearly indicates that families are a priority to God. He established the family as a means to reproduce His nature throughout the generations. The family unit begins in Genesis and continues throughout the New Testament. God views us as individuals connected to families. Family order and function are important because they teach us purpose and meaning in life. The Old Testament reflects God's use of the family as the means to set up His kingdom here on earth. He made some families priests, some farmers, and some builders; but no matter their calling, each family played a role in the community of God.

Eventually, the family unit gave birth to the Messiah. The genealogy of Jesus holds a place of great prominence in the first chapter of the gospel of Matthew. One reason that chapter gives an entire account of Jesus' lineage is that God's desire was to reflect the spiritual heritage of Christ. Families and their heritage are a big deal to God.

Our family upbringing engrains patterns in us that are rooted in the flesh but impact us body, soul, and spirit. The training we receive at home during childhood establishes the foundation for the way we act, believe, think, speak, and feel. We are either trained to live according to God's laws and principles or influenced to live in ungodly ways. In essence, our training brings blessings or curses upon our families.

If our parents, grandparents, or other extended family raised us in the absence of the blessing, then we may go searching for the blessing outside of God's kingdom. Of those who are searching, some will land in the church—only to find more struggles because there is family dysfunction in the church, too. For instance, if we come from a controlling family system, we will most often find ourselves in controlling church relationships within the church because that kind of situation is what we are drawn to. Likewise, if we come from a performance based family system where love was measured by perfection and success, then we will find ourselves drawn to a church that operates on those same beliefs. In cases such as these, the church can produce more inner conflict and further spiritual turmoil by perpetuating the family patterns that produce curses on our lives.

The family is a powerful environment for shaping our understanding of God, self, and others. The traits we develop in childhood will carry over into adulthood as we form new relationships that affirm our beliefs. I find it no surprise that when we dig around in a person's family background, we find information that leads to causes of that person's current problems.

Curses pass from generation to generation in a number of ways. We receive the spiritual heritage of our forefathers whether we like it or not. Like a waterfall, that heritage proceeds downhill to the land below. We may choose to divorce our family, but it does not rid us of the traits that we receive from them genetically or spiritually. We can receive curses through the genetic code of our bloodline.

When we are first conceived, both our father and mother give us a gene that determines our blood type and reproduces a genetic formation for our blood.[2] The blood in our bodies carries with it a vast number of cells that make up the life of our body. Therefore, if our parents' blood is contaminated with a disease, chances are, the disease will be passed on to us. A situation such as this could create a vast number of possible health concerns. Yet the truth is, once we submit our lives to Christ, His blood cleanses us from all unrighteousness. That is good news! Not only can our physical heritage be changed—for instance, disease is not righteous; it can be cleansed out of the blood (which I will cover later on)—but our spiritual heritage can be changed as well.

As you can see, the training we receive from our parents, grandparents, other extended family, or guardian opens the door for us to receive a wealth of understanding or a bucketful of lies. If our parents motivated us with threats and violence, then we learned to live in fear; but if our parents used positive reinforcement and conditioned us with affirmation, we learned to respond to love. Training involves teaching and empowering someone to respond to life in specific ways. If the way you were raised caused you to develop a fear mentality, let me remind you of what Paul said to Timothy, his beloved disciple: "God did not give us a spirit, or a mentality, of fear, but one of love, power, and a sound mind" (2 Tim. 1:7). This scripture gives you the option to break free from the unhealthy dictates you learned from your parents.

The enemy may be very good at trying to keep us deceived with the thought that our problems are just due to the way we are and are not related to our forefathers' sins. However, the truth is that there's a way to break free and separate ourselves from the ungodly influences of our past generations.

From Cursed to Blessed

Through the life, death, and resurrection of Christ, God made complete provision for our sin, our sinfulness, and our propensity to sin. The blessing of God's atonement, which was His offering made for our sin, offers us a new life. This new life opens the door for us to be part of a new family. We get to be in the family of God because He made a way for us to be a member. We are grafted into this family birthright by faith (Rom. 11:23) Once we are in, we get to be blessed, because God, the Father of our new family, doesn't curse His own kids; He blesses them. We get to overcome because He overcame—no questions asked. These benefits are all ours if we will receive them and apply them to our lives.

I find that, as believers, many of us have only a superficial understanding of our spiritual heritage in Christ. Specifically, we do not understand God's provision for His own kids. As a result, many of us are sick and dying. We lack understanding because previous generations have not provided it, nor has it been a priority. We emphasize things like education, marriage, career, and location when it comes to finding the blessings of life, but these are not God's order for finding His blessings.

Receiving God's blessings involves learning to submit to Him by faith. Abraham was a man who learned to have great faith. His life is an excellent example of breaking away from a generation of unrighteous people and becoming righteous through faith. The book of Genesis records how God called Abraham to follow Him to a new place away from his father's people. Abraham set out, not knowing where he was going (Gen. 12:1). Later, by faith he received the promise of God—that he would have a son in his old age.

During the unfolding of this story, Abraham learned to walk with God by faith, but it was not an overnight process. The promise given to him, that he would have a son who would represent the people of God, took many years to happen. Abraham struggled to believe and receive the promise because he and his wife, Sarah, were old. Because of his fear and insecurity, he tried to take matters into his own hands along the way, and he ended up creating many problems for himself. But he matured in the process by accepting God's promise as true.

Paul records in Romans that, by faith, Abraham learned to speak things into being that did not exist in the natural (Rom. 4:17). The promise manifested as a result of Abraham's learning to exchange his weakness for the strength of God. And not only did Abraham eventually receive the promise of a son, his life was also rich and full because of the blessings of God.

When we become born again, we have the same spiritual heritage as Abraham (Gal. 3:29). We're going to see next that, because of this rich heritage, we can walk away from curses such as sickness, poverty, divorce, and infertility, as we apply God's Word (by speaking it) to each curse and remove it from our lives. God is interested in our becoming totally curse-free and living a life of freedom as His representatives on the earth. If you were to pick players for a sporting event, would you pick the ones who are going to lose or the ones who are going to win? God wants us to win, so He changes losers into winners. That is what the gospel is all about.

Breaking Free

Breaking curses is like undressing after being out in a very cold snow-storm. We take off the extra layers of clothing because they keep us too warm after coming inside. Sometimes curses come off like rubber boots that are hard to remove because they are so tight that they seem to be permanent; but each piece of burdensome clothing must be removed if we are going to find true peace and happiness.

The power to break destructive cycles comes from one source—the same power we use to overcome sin and the nature of sin—Jesus Christ, the risen Son of God. Yet power does not come because of a one-time declaration to yield to Jesus. To remove every generational sin, we must apply both the Word of God and the blood of Christ to the curses in our lives (Rev. 12:11). We apply the blood the same way we apply the Word—by speaking it over ourselves and others. When we do, God removes the curses off our lives just as He did for the Israelites in the Old Testament.

If you recall, God told them to smear the blood of a lamb on the doorposts of their homes during the first Passover. The death angel[3] came and killed the firstborn of every household, but he could not touch the people inside the homes where the lambs' blood was applied to their doors. The "destroyer" had to pass over those houses. The blood bought the Israelites freedom from death, as well as deliverance from over four hundred years of Egyptian bondage (Ex. 12:21–23, 30–41).

This powerful event illustrates the nature of God regarding sin and its consequences. He provides the blood of the Lamb for covering our sin; we apply that blood to the door of our hearts by faith, knowing that we are cleansed from our iniquities and empowered to overcome all sin, including the sin of our forefathers.

We can pronounce our freedom from the destructive cycles of our ancestors as we confess their known iniquities, their patterns of sin, before God. That should be our goal. The blueprint for our declaration is found in the Old Testament in Ezra 9, Nehemiah 2 and 9, and Daniel 9. We are taking the responsibility to renounce the iniquity of the generations before us, but we are not taking responsibility for someone else's sin. We are confessing the cycle of evil and seeking God to end the destruction. We are looking to God to intervene in our life and family, and lift the darkness off of us.

Confession is a powerful tool that leads to healing and restoration. The apostle James said that confessing our faults to one another brings healing (James 5:16). Admission of sin releases its power over us, but the sin we keep in the dark grows. Family secrets breed many problems, like mold growing on the back wall of a refrigerator.

The process of breaking generational curses not only involves confession, but forgiveness, renouncing, repenting, and exchanging the old patterns of cursed living with a new model of living that is founded on the Bible:

- We *forgive* those who committed sin against God, others, or self. Forgiveness is releasing someone of a debt against us.

- We *renounce* behaviors, words spoken against others or God. Renouncing involves falling out of agreement with one party and coming into agreement with another party. We break agreement with any of our forefathers' commitments to Satan and his practices, and come into agreement with God.

▶ We *repent* for the sin of the past. Repenting involves changing our direction. Our parents may have walked in rebellion toward God, but we choose to walk in submission to Him.

▶ Finally, we *exchange* all curses, all the consequence of sin, with the blessing of God. We replace the kingdom of darkness with the kingdom of light. This means, if we are living according to the lies of the enemy and covering the sin of the past in any area of our life, we expose it to the light of God's Word. We confront the darkness in our family; we no longer walk in it. We tear down the structures and beliefs that are idolatrous. We take time to remove all strongholds in our life that give the devil access to us and to our family.

This process takes work and a willingness to persevere through it, but power for overcoming sin and destructive cycles comes as we continue to say yes to God daily. Every day we have to receive from Him the power to live. His power, rightly appropriated, brings intervention in our life. He gives us authority to overcome because He came into the earth as a real man and paved the way for us to do so. We'll cover the subject of our authority more later on, but here's the key: We must have God's Spirit at work in us—the infilling of the Holy Spirit.

The Holy Spirit is the power of God that enables us to do things we couldn't do on our own. For instance, He gives us strength to overcome the generational issues in our lives. Some say that the devil is our adversary and that his plan is to perpetuate the cycle of familial sin in our lives. I could not agree more. Specifically, he is going to come against you and seek to destroy you through one of your generational weaknesses. If fear was a big issue in your family, then Satan would use fear to come against you. The same principle applies to addictions. Alcoholics become alcoholics because they are spiritually predisposed to the problem. The enemy sets us up to give in to these predispositions in moments of weakness; then we become caught in the cycle.

It is now a well-known fact that you do not have to drink alcohol or do drugs to be an addict. Addiction comes in many socially acceptable forms these days; a person may be addicted to caffeine, sugar, comfort food, work, exercise, or sex. Many addicts are exposed to family dynamics that train them in a particular lifestyle of addiction.

So if we expect generational patterns of iniquities and the ensuing curses that follow them to be changed, we must rise up within our families and take a stand. Taking a stand involves facing the obvious sin that no one else is willing to face. The need to do so is quite evident to me whenever I conduct a funeral. Without fail, the family gathers, most of its members wanting to believe the best about the deceased. But if their thoughts were truly communicated, they would tell a different story. Many relatives walk by the casket, knowing the deceased's struggles all too well—because they face the same struggles every day in their own lives. The question is, what are they doing to get rid of those struggles?

It is clearly a matter of what quality of life we seek to live. Shall we wink at sin and hope the death angel passes over our door? Or shall we know for sure where we stand with God? I want peace in my life, and more than that, I want to know I stood for the right thing. Isn't that what you want?

You may have been born into a Christian family, but be careful; just because your family appears acceptable to society doesn't mean there are not curses lurking at the door. You must take a stand and allow God to purge you from all uncleanness and unrighteousness, beginning with surrendering your life to Him. It takes courage to break free from generational sin, but you only stand to gain when you put away the iniquity of your forefathers.

The blessings of God are for those who are willing to take hold of them by applying the Word to their lives. If someone had left us an inheritance in a bank, at some point we would have to go draw the money out in order to benefit from it. In the same way, if we expect to draw on our spiritual inheritance, we must make room for it by cleaning out the curses and replacing them with the blessings.

Prayer:

Father, I pray that all the sins and iniquities of past generations be forgiven and released from my life. Leave no stone left unturned. Expose all evil. Reveal all sources of sin and every iniquity so that I may confess them and be forgiven.

Father, I recognize and take responsibility for the iniquity of past generations and for all of their unrighteousness. I ask You to wipe the slate clean from rebellion, idolatry, occultism, bitterness, unbelief, pride, rejection, envy, jealousy, hatred, immorality, unclean actions, and any other sexual sins—all forms of iniquity that I know of, as well as any that I am unaware of. I ask that these sins be purged from my bloodline and that every curse be broken in the name of Jesus Christ. I believe that the shed blood of Jesus gives me power and authority to end the cycle of sin in this generation today.

Let Your great blessings replace the curses. I now exchange disease, poverty, infertility, divorce, alcoholism, and all other curses for the blessings of health, wealth, fertility, a strong marriage and family, and fruit in every other field of my life. I pray in the name of Jesus Christ, expecting to receive. Amen.

CHAPTER 8

"HE RESTORES MY SOUL"

A Transformation of Character

AS WE DISCUSSED IN CHAPTER 7, THE DELIVERANCE PROCESS is an integral step toward greater freedom in Christ. In fact, deliverance from demonic oppression can bring mental, emotional, and physical relief, in addition to clarity of mind. However, for those of us who are deeply wounded in our souls, there is a need to go further still. For that reason, we will open the door to see how our souls can be healed and transformed from brokenness to wholeness. This chapter will deal with how to replenish what the enemy has stolen from us. We will learn how to move beyond a shame-based personality by receiving a genuine cleansing touch from God. Only His touch can remove shame, deposit deep and abiding security, heal memories, and bring freedom to our souls.

Born-again Christians suffer just as other people do. We face trials and difficulties as a part of living in an imperfect, fallen world (Gen. 3). The apostle Paul said that believers inherit both the blessings of salvation and the persecution of the world (Rom. 8:17). But we have something the world doesn't have—the promises of God.

God's promises are granted to us by His grace, through which we receive the power to overcome our earthly struggles. It is interesting to note that as Jesus was preparing to leave this world, He prayed His disciples would be preserved while remaining in it (John 17:15). Notice He did not pray that they be removed from the world or the effects of the world—only that they be protected. Likewise, we, as present-day believers, must endure hardship (2 Tim. 2:3), knowing that we have a Protector who meets us in our suffering and promises to lead us to restoration if we will follow Him.

Now, there are some who teach a pain-free gospel that eliminates all trials in life, often mixing biblical fact and psychological insight. I believe this kind of message alters the point of living the Christian life from serving and following after Christ to running from, medicating, or completely ignoring the darkness in our soul. These messengers want us to believe that we should not have to experience the pressures of life or embrace the reality of suffering in the world, or that we can submerge ourselves in the ecstasy of profound spirituality to such a degree that it will eliminate suffering altogether. Instead, their message should be strengthening us to walk through and overcome hardship as we learn to live in a real world.

According to them, faith is no longer the trail that leads to peace and contentment, but the vehicle that we use to rearrange our circumstances in an effort to avoid suffering. This kind of teaching pushes a gospel that sounds as though God were our servant instead of our being His. The result of believing such an idea is that we become numb to the reality that we live in a world where evil is prevalent and persecution is real.

No matter what practice or combination of practices we use to relieve or eliminate our suffering, the truth is that there is no overnight transformation or "gos-pill" to take for instant relief from what lies within our souls. (The miraculous intervention of God's supernatural touch comes in extraordinary ways, but there is still a need for deeper change.) The alleviation of physical symptoms does not rule out the need for sanctification. For example, I received a major touch from God that released me from the infirmity of hepatitis, but

I still needed a deeper work in my soul to be whole. The profound process of repentance and release of the past continued the healing and took over two years. To this day, I continue to go deeper as I allow God to remove and replace the things I have stored in my heart that don't belong there. The healing touch of God is the only thing that can deliver us and set us free.

Can You Really Be Free?

Can we enter the deep recesses of our souls, where the reality of darkness is often more consuming than the evidence of Christ, and examine the condition of our self-centeredness? Is God really capable of handling all the junk stored in the closet and attic spaces of our hearts and minds? Or would it just be simpler to play pretend and get on with being a good Christian? Can we really change?

Change is possible if you are willing to go through the process and allow God to perform it. In other words, change is only possible as an extended work of His grace. Change does come with a price, however. Of course, Jesus paid the ultimate price, but change will cost you, too. You must give up the control of your life and yield to the deep, inner work of the Holy Spirit. I have prayed the prayer to be transformed by God many times, but taking steps to walk out that transformation has required a new level of faith and dependence on Him because my flesh wants to remain independent and in charge of my life.

The truth is that God desires to pour out His mercy on us, but we cannot receive it unless we are open to change. He wants to shed light on all of our darkness, but we must be willing to learn to walk in the light. Our goal is often pain relief, but God's goal is much deeper—the transformation of our lives. Our heavenly Father wants to change us into people who truly reflect His character, that we may be noble, unswerving, bold, and courageous, even when faced with life's realities.

Religion and spirituality based on pretense do not equip us to be overcomers; rather, they enable us to live as victims. The Lord, on the other hand, enables us to endure in the midst of struggle, stare hardship in the face, witness corruption and evil in the world, and experience His healing if we face the dread of disease. Though at times we may feel overwhelmed, if we will rely on Him, we will come out in the end, unshaken in our faith and determined to press on in life—a life that exemplifies His power to overcome. (Remember, through Christ's atonement, we can overcome.) This route is the road less traveled, the narrow gate spoken of by Christ in the Bible.

> *Go in through the narrow gate, for wide is the gate and broad is the way that leads to destruction, and many there are who go in through it. Because narrow is the gate and constricted is the way which leads to life, and there are few who find it.*
> MATTHEW 7:13–14

The narrow way happens to be the only road to true transformation of our beliefs and character. Gaining hints of the potential freedom we can have by traveling this less-sought-after path motivates us to go on, making the thought of returning to our former life of torment simply unthinkable. The concept of suffering begins to take on new meaning as we begin to live the reality of giving up our lives so we can gain His in return. Now, this kind of transformation is worth any pain!

You may be reading this book, looking for answers to your pain. I am familiar with that journey. I empathize with you if you are working out issues of suffering in your life. I deeply respect the agony and fear involved in facing yourself and the throbbing inside your heart. You may even feel confusion about how God is going to heal and set you free. Maybe you have totally given up. Do not buy into the lie that God will not meet you in your troubles.

Let me encourage you with this: God has not given up on you. Your life is not over; the end has not yet come. God will not let you go. Your Deliverer is standing ready and willing to set you free from the anguish and anxiety brought on in your suffering. God wants to take you by the hand and lead you into a safe place where there is healing from the inside out.

The *narrow path* is the process of character transformation that leads to this healing of the soul. Sometimes we need to grow up, and sometimes we need healing within our hearts to aid the growth. This process is what Christ was referring to when He talked about the broad and narrow paths of life. The broad one leads to destruction because many of us are unwilling to surrender our hearts to God. As a result, we miss out on the blessing of God's healing, transforming power.

I met a man once who requested my help because he was struggling with a disease he could not find a cure for. He had spent several million dollars seeking out numerous types of treatment, but to no avail. Out of desperation, he inquired what I did to help people. When I told him, his response was that he was not interested in submitting His life to Jesus Christ.

If we are not willing to walk the narrow path that leads to life, then we must be willing to face the life we create for ourselves. I cannot stress this point strongly enough. Some sick people whom I meet (like this man) desire healing, but they struggle to want God. Actually, we often want the benefits of God but secretly hope the requirements are not too severe. Yet God's covenant is clear regarding the hierarchy of submission—He is the leader and we must be willing followers, meaning that He is the boss, not vice versa. His way of leading is not to force us into submission but to invite us to a place of surrender. He is not like the evil dictator who crushes His opponents after battle. Upon laying down our arms, God restores us and mends our wounds.

Let Go, Fall Back, and Trust God

Making ourselves ready for this journey requires a deep level of surrender. The very thing we have struggled to do our whole life is trust others. Trust is a prerequisite for releasing the emotional bondage of the past. Trust is like repelling off the side of a mountain cliff by leaning over the edge and falling backward. We tie the rope tightly around us and know that as we lean back, there is a short distance in which we will fall. That distance is known as the "mental edge." We fall back until the rope catches us and our body is perpendicular with the face of the rock. We must trust that the one supporting us will not let go.

This example parallels the process we must go through with God. Only when we take the risk and trust Him do we find out that He is more than able to handle us if we fall. Trust is not built until we take a risk, but for some, we experience a mental block when trying to full surrender to God, even though we know we need His help.

Many of us run through a cycle something like this: We go see our pastor, hoping he or she can pray our pain away. That doesn't work, so the pastor sends us to a counselor, in hopes the counselor can help us manage our pain. The counselor cannot fix us, so we're sent to a doctor; maybe he or she can heal our pain. But the doctor cannot heal our pain, so we're sent to a pharmacist to get medication; perhaps the pharmacist's medicine will numb our pain—and it does temporarily.

I am by no means implying that you should not seek help and guidance from any of these professionals. They can and will be instrumental in guiding you through the healing process. But they cannot do it for you. My point is that all professionals, including myself, are limited. You cannot depend on us for something that only you can do with God. We can only help you go so far in your journey.

Only God can restore a wounded soul that is aching in pain. His way of restoration strengthens our spirit and heals our bodies. His touch may come through one of His servants, but if we are expecting people to do it for us, we are in for a rude awakening. So, let go, fall back, and trust God. He is able to support you, because He created you and knows exactly how to fix what is broken.

How do you trust God, whom you cannot see and struggle to feel? You start by simply asking Him for help. Admit you cannot make this journey by yourself. Express your heart to Him. Ask Him to reveal Himself to you. Listen for His voice in your heart. Lean on others who have been down this road for support and guidance. You are not required to fix yourself, only to surrender your life to Him. Letting God take the lead is the best thing you could ever do for yourself. We were not designed to be in control. We were created to be dependent. God shows up as we lean upon Him and invite Him to bring healing and restoration, because He is faithful to His Word.

When I first started this process, I learned that I received more from God if I listened to His voice in my heart than if I shouted out my thoughts to Him. I had been taught that prayer and interaction with God were about learning how to make your requests known. But I found out that prayer goes much deeper than that—I had to learn how to hear His voice and receive His direction. Prayer is more like learning to absorb God and interact with Him. A crisis mentality, which most of us have during sickness or emergencies, focuses on putting out fires and obtaining quick results. But God is not moved by our desperation for results. He is moved by the man or woman who wants to have a relationship with Him. Relationship is built around yielding and receiving, not pushing and pulling. The only scary part to this process, as we saw earlier, is that we lose control of our lives.

Those of us who grew up in a family that controlled our every move with anger and fear will find it tough as an adult to release the steering wheel of our lives to another. It is not our nature to trust. We do not want to be vulnerable and ask for help. We want to keep running our life ourselves, dreaming that someday it will be all better. In other words, we want medicine, but we want to take it on our own terms.

Our unwillingness to surrender often takes on the appearance of self-determination, making us look like we are trying hard to do what is right. But, believe me, no one is taking our situation seriously. I speak from experience because I played that game for years, and I know what a deception it is. Our struggle is not that others aren't giving us a break; it is that we are unwilling to trust and do not want others to tell us what to do. Every time we get close to resolving our pain, we run from it because we are forced to look at our own responsibility. We cannot expect God to push our will out of the way and heal us in spite of our stubbornness—He does not work that way. Remember, He created us with a free will to choose. He wants to help us, but requires that we lay down our will so that He can be in charge.

The evidence of trusting God is peace in our hearts, regardless of the circumstances. Trusting Him means we resolve the fear of losing control and we stand ready to face any storm that shows itself on the horizon. Trust produces a sense of security in us, and allows God to move on our behalf. In the end, He will prove Himself reliable. Paul said it like this, "If God is for us, who can be against us?" (Rom. 8:31).

Your Pain Is Your Gain

How many times have I attempted to go down this path? Taking a heartfelt look into my soul has been a lifelong process. At times I felt like I was going through open-heart surgery. The emotional pain was so deep and heavy at certain points, I felt I might physically collapse and wondered if I could go on another minute. The emotional weight that accompanies the wounds of childhood and the traumas of life can be excruciating. The pain from these wounds had compounded throughout my life, and because they remained internalized, I suffered serious consequences. However, one truth I will no longer deny—the trail of pain in my past will not order the steps of my future.

Let me pause for a second and tell you the truth about working through the deep wounds of the soul. It does not have to take a lifetime, nor does it have to hold us in bondage our entire life. I know others who have received grace and moved on with their lives just as I have. I believe that is God's heart for all His children. I think God puts people in our lives, leads us to places, and opens the door for the cavalry to come to our aid, but we must recognize it and yield to our Redeemer. Otherwise, the presence of freedom becomes a source of frustration and cynicism.

Liberation fuels anger in the heart of a man bent on rebelling. That is the reason my process had been so ugly and so tough—I had been unwilling to yield my will to God. In the past, my mode of operation had been to fight it. Nevertheless, I discovered that my greatest weakness can be an asset because the power of the unwillingness, once corrected, becomes a force of will to believe and stand for truth. My brokenness is now His glorification, and for that I am very grateful. That is why I have dedicated my life to giving away this gospel of redemption.

If we expect the ache in our heart to be removed without pain, we are in a delusion. It is going to hurt. The reality of the pain we feel in our broken heart is an indicator that it must be released. To get rid of this agony will require work on our part. It does not just leave. We must prepare ourselves for freedom. If we were captured and taken prisoner, in order to escape, we would first have to get ourselves ready mentally. This is also true when it comes to inner healing and releasing the wounds of the past.

The depth of pain is dependent upon how long you hang onto the reigns after being thrown off from the course. If you grit your teeth and refuse God's gentle moving, then the pain is going to submerge deeper and deeper into your soul. It is better not to be bitter. It is a more excellent thing to yield and allow the Lord to restore you.

The pain principle is the most powerful force in life when it comes to inspiring change. In fact, there is no greater motivation. We will do almost anything to get out of pain. The culture we live in is rooted in this principle of escaping of pain. For instance, two core motivations in today's society are (1) avoiding what causes pain and (2) finding what brings pleasure. This approach to pain is consistent with every generation. We say, "Count me in," if it brings happiness and "Count me out," if it brings suffering.

Yet God uses the pain in our lives to teach us, although I have made it clear that He is *not* the author of it. He does not allow us to suffer just for the sake of suffering. He uses the course of tribulations that we all face to teach us to overcome. The very story of the gospel of Christ is a message of triumph directed to all the people of this world. The Father sent His Son into the world to provide a real means of victory for His people. Jesus' pain and suffering and resurrection from death give us hope. Our pain and suffering can be exchanged for His blessings, including healing and restoration.

Finding purpose in our hurts can lead to transformation and cause our pain to be our gain.

The most vulnerable hour in the life of Jesus was when He went to the Garden of Gethsemane to pray, prior to His betrayal. Remember, He went there to prepare Himself for what was to come, and the disciples were to be doing the same. He entered the garden, a familiar place, and told the disciples to stay at the entrance, but He took three of them with Him as He went a little farther. Then He asked the three to tarry there, drew even farther into the garden, and prayed to the Father. The positioning of the disciples is important to us because each group of people represented the invitation to deeper levels of intimacy with God, by their placement in the garden (Matt. 26:36–39).

While praying, Jesus revealed that He was troubled in His soul. This troubling was so deep that it eventually produced sweat in the form of drops of blood (Luke 22:44). This mind-altering, body-shaking, soul-wrenching emotional pain was the weight of our sin. Jesus knew that taking our sin would ultimately separate Him from the Father, and He knew it was coming—but He also knew that He had to go all the way to the cross in order to fulfill the purpose of Messiah.

His agony was so great there in the garden that He needed the assistance of an angel from heaven to strengthen Him (v. 43). The fact that He needed aid from an angel allows us to relate to Him as a man. Needing supernatural help was even a requirement for the Son of God. That should encourage us in our own journey. Nevertheless, prayer and submission are the keys to His success in obedience to the Father. He said, "Not My will, but Yours be done" (v. 42). It is in this exchange that the real man Jesus found the real power of God to go to the cross.

Jesus prayed the same prayer, not once or twice but three times. That gives me hope. How many times have I prayed the same prayer, wondering if it helped at all? The captors of Christ came for Him, but what they didn't realize was that He was responsible for turning the story of the human race in a different direction that night in the Garden of Gethsemane. He reversed the curse and yielded to the Father so that now the very same opportunity is made possible for us. Remember, all things are possible for those who believe (Mark 9:23).

Experience the Goodness of God

There is no greater demonstration of perfect love than the portrayal of God's mercy for us in giving His Son to be a ransom for our sinfulness. God arranged all of history to create an opportunity for His love to be real for all of mankind. He offers us His love with an invitation to experience the exchange of our misery for the gift of life in Christ. You have before you the greatest opportunity of your lifetime. You get to lay down a life of suffering in exchange for a life of fulfillment. That is a reason to get out of bed every morning.

God often uses others to initiate the inner healing process in our lives, as He did for me through one of my dearest friends, Clay McLean (singer, songwriter, Bible teacher, and a true man of God). What God did for me, He can do for you. We can have hope for inner healing because we have a loving, gentle, heavenly Father who is poised to embrace us in our hurt and anguish of soul. His soothing nature provides a sense of safety and security to the shattered heart; He desires to draw us close and hold us until our pain subsides and we discover His reality. The Father loves people and desires that we all know Him. *Knowing Him* means inviting Him to be part of every area of our life, even the darkest recesses of our soul.

The reflection of God as Father can be seen in His relationship with Jesus, the Son. Christ is a mirror image of the heart of the Father. His life, His ministry, His relationships with people, His willingness to serve others, His strength, and His obedience are all traits of God. It is said that we become like those we spend time with. That concept is certainly true of the Son, who demonstrated the character of the Father on earth.

Many times Christ left the presence of others to receive from His Father. Jesus mentioned more than once that His life was one with the Father (John 17:22–23), and there was and is an abiding unity between the Father and the Son. Out of that unity came the anointing for Christ to eliminate suffering. He did it every place He went, even in His last hour as He forgave one of the thieves on the cross next to His (Luke 23:40–43).

This offers us great hope. During His last hours on earth, Christ prayed for His followers that they might be one with the Father (John 17:11). Jesus willingly offered up His life for sacrifice, knowing that He was making a way for us to know the Father. He spent His agonizing time on the cross, knowing that, through His sacrifice, sinners around the world would be able to have eternal life and receive the loving touch of the Father here on earth.

The most masculine demonstration of perfect love was the death of Christ. True masculinity is about embracing weakness, not prancing around boasting about testosterone levels. Jesus' embrace of our state of sinfulness and pitiful weakness was motivated by the Father's love and embrace of an inept people who could not free themselves.

Our heavenly Father could not stand by and watch us suffer without extending Himself to meet us in our real pain. Our motto at this ministry came from that truth: "He sent His Son, a real man, into the real world to deliver us from our real suffering." The Father's plan is that we might exchange the darkness in our soul for the light of His love. He faithfully executed every action, preparing the way for the Son of man to open the door to His unending acceptance.

I believe that there is no more important scripture than John 3:16. It tells the whole story.

> For God so loved the world that He gave His only-begotten Son, that whoever believes in Him should not perish but have everlasting life.

The Father promises to restore us to right relationship with Him if we yield to the plan. Trusting the Father is about learning to be a son or a daughter.[1] I had a hard time with that concept because my relationship with my dad was so troubling most of my life that, for me, trusting anyone masculine and in authority was like needing to visit the dentist—I might have known I needed to go but would put it off until I couldn't stand the pain another hour.

We cannot fully experience the goodness of God until we allow Him to love us. Unlike the limited love of our earthly fathers, God the Father's love toward us is perfect. He reaches for us with perfect motivation, only to heal us and establish us as His children.

Healing the Broken Heart

If you have hurt in your heart, it will be necessary to receive the Father's love to mend it. I find that many of us have a gap in our faith when it comes to receiving God's love. We acknowledge the need for His love, but we struggle to know it for ourselves because there is a point of separation between us and God. The best way to describe it is to say that the relationship is awkward. We want to experience God's love, but because we do not feel it, we doubt it. We want to know God but find Him unapproachable.

I have found that the point of disconnect between us and God is derived from our perception. Our understanding of Him is limited. We do not know His nature, so it is hard for us to believe that His love is real. We tend to see God as we view our earthly fathers. Our relationship with Abba is a reflection of our relationship with Daddy. A relationship with Dad that was complicated and a source of pain produces doubt that we can have a relationship with God that is founded on love and acceptance.

The typical reason that we struggle to know God's love for ourselves is that it is hard for us to get beyond what we experienced in our relationship with our earthly fathers. If we hold onto the hurt of our childhood, then we will not be able to receive our heavenly Father's love. A broken heart caused by wounding in our primary years often-times leaves a very deep pain. It seems we have ways of holding onto that pain and submerging it beneath our attempts to find success and happiness. Nevertheless, the inner pain of childhood, teenage years, or adulthood must be faced for the sake of our recovery and sanity.

Most of the time, our hearts get broken because someone else inflicts pain on us. We must release the person who is responsible for the wound; otherwise, we will perpetuate the cycle of victimization in our lives. The scent of a victim will draw perpetrators to hurt us again, and we may even be oblivious as to why this cycle continues in our lives.

On occasion these wounds are self-inflicted. Sometimes our hearts are broken because we have hurt ourselves. Yes, it is possible for us to injure ourselves; the emotional pain can be self-inflicted. Often it happens because we are trying to produce love or become lovable to others. We desperately want the approval of others and will do anything to get it, even if it requires that we subject ourselves to personal pain and loss. The important thing to remember is, whether our wound was self-inflicted or caused by someone else, a broken heart can only be repaired by the embrace of our loving heavenly Father.

I found that God replaced the void left by the difficult relationship I had with my dad. One major thing God did was use godly men to embrace, nurture, and support me. All of these people were unselfish and supportive in their willingness to see me develop and grow as a person. Learning to become a son was a tough thing for me, but I thank God, my heavenly Father, for the God-given dads He placed in my life.

Let's face it; human fathers are imperfect, including the one writing these pages. For one thing, we do not always know how to love properly. Some fathers are unable to love because they were loved imperfectly themselves. I know that my dad wanted to be a different man. I saw him try to work hard and provide for his family. He wanted to do the right thing, but he was not aware of the spiritual battle he faced. He was controlled by the forces of addiction and fear, and his life was greatly tormented. I can remember as a young boy many times wanting to go to him, but feeling afraid that he would reject me or get angry with me about my weakness. So I adopted a pattern in my life of thinking things were always my fault, because it was not safe to bring up issues of weakness in my home.

I visit with a lot of people who report a similar childhood, and through my own experience I'm able to tell them that the broken heart is mended as we receive God's words of healing into the recesses of stored pain within our souls. He gently opens the door and touches us where it hurts emotionally. He releases each painful trauma and the memory associated with it. This process unfolds as we learn to practice listening and healing prayer, which we'll look at in a moment. First, I want to share something else with you about God's healing love.

Become Holdable

Our loving heavenly Father makes it safe to face the pain in our lives. Receiving His love is a process that begins as we come to know Him. Eventually it grows deeper as we yield our wounds to Him. He embraces us and holds us until we are okay—that is, if we let Him.

My youngest daughter, Darcy, taught me this lesson when she was about eighteen months old. One day she was playing and having a good time, and I scooped her up off the floor, hoping for a big hug and kiss. But Darcy was "unholdable." She was not interested; so instead, she squirmed out of my arms and back to the floor. Later on that evening, the Lord spoke to me in my heart that sometimes we, as adult Christians, are the same way. We are unwilling to allow Him to embrace us and hold us; our heavenly Father wants to hold us, but we are unholdable.

The process of overcoming our internal wounds is a process of becoming holdable. God will hold us until the pain is gone. How does He hold us? He uses people to embrace us in our most vulnerable situations. We confess our pain, and God uses those who stand with us to walk through the pain alongside us as it surfaces.

God guides us in very practical ways to work out these situations with others; His Word and His ways are very practical. Ironically, God often uses other wounded people who have been through similar situations to help us through this process. I call them "wounded healers." The goal is our freedom and a deeper dependence upon the Lord. This time is very powerful because all the bad memories that have loomed over us for so many years disintegrate in the presence of God.

"Where two or three are gathered together in My name, there I am in their midst."

MATTHEW 18:20

Again, through the process of inner healing, God leads us in releasing the past by the work of His Spirit inside of us. He guides us each step of the way, many times with the help of experienced ministers. I find that this healing process happens for most people in layers, or stages. God, in His infinite wisdom, knows that when there are many layers of hurt from many years of pain, we could not possibly handle the release of it all at once. So, ultimately, the process takes time.

Darlena and I had worked for many years on ourselves, a process that began in our twenties. So when it came time to get into the depths of the soil of our soul, we did not have much further to dig. After that time, we spent two years of our lives focused almost solely on the restoration of our souls.

Remember, we cannot put a timeframe on the healing process. Becoming holdable requires time and patience.

Working through Internal Wounds

You may be struggling with the thought of digging around in the past and stirring up things that have been put to bed long ago. Just because time has passed does not guarantee that these wounds are laid aside. Test it for yourself. Are you still being controlled by memories of the past? When you think about certain experiences or spend time with others who represent your hurt, are painful memories triggered? Are you acting out of your past, or are you living from today forward?

I once saw a man beating his wife in a parking lot, and it activated a deep hurt in me from my past that caused me to jump out of my truck with the intention of evening the score. However, a friend I was with jarred my attention and persuaded me to calm down. Unfortunately, by the time I composed myself enough to offer help in a rational way, the man and his wife had already left the lot. Situations like these are signs we need healing in the damaged areas of our hearts.

In ministry, we take our model for working through the internal wounds of the past from a scriptural principle seen throughout the Bible. God often used past failures and traumas to teach His people how to alleviate suffering. For example, the Psalms are reflections of the emotions, thoughts, and expressions of people who sought God's blessings and learned to walk beyond the weakness of human struggle. Each Psalm reflects an expression to God regarding the ordinary circumstances of life. Let's look at a few of them.

> *He restores my soul; He leads me in paths of righteousness for His name's sake.*
>
> PSALM 23:3

> *I said, Jehovah, be merciful to me; heal my soul; for I have sinned against You.*
>
> PSALM 41:4

> *He heals the broken-hearted, and binds up their wounds.*
>
> PSALM 147:3

All of these writings address the need and desire for a wounded heart to be restored. Moses wrote in the book of Exodus that God revealed Himself as Jehovah Rapha—the God who heals us[2] (15:26). In addition, Isaiah prophesied that the Messiah would be someone who released us from our grief and sorrow (Isa. 53:4). The apostle John wrote in his exhortation in his third epistle that he wished above all things that we find good health, including health in our souls (3 John 2). Inner healing is a common theme among the writers of the New Testament. Luke recorded that Jesus stood before a synagogue of people and proclaimed that His ministry was dedicated to healing the brokenhearted (Luke 4:18). John 14:26 refers to the Holy Spirit as the Comforter. These attributes reflect the nature of God to heal. As you can see, He takes our wounds from the past very seriously.

At times the process of healing the soul may need to include deep ministry. In case you are not familiar with this, here is a brief description of a procedure that may take a number of ministry sessions, lasting over an extended period of time. This method for releasing the burdens is simple and yet very delicate, but anyone seeking ministry must first submit to it.

We start by walking someone who is ready for the healing to begin through a time of prayer. Afterward, we proceed by investigating the experience that continues to weigh upon them as a burden. This part involves key questions to gain insight into the struggle from the past. It may comprise a number of circumstances, but it is important to note that the investigation process is about helping a person connect the pain of the past to a current struggle.

We do that by focusing on the memory of that event, all the while being mindful of the presence of the Holy Spirit—but we do not create memories or suggest scenarios. Ministers must be careful not to suggest insight or create experiences. Doing so only causes the person confusion and more pain. Instead, ministers need to allow the Holy Spirit to bring up the key issues through the person receiving ministry.

The goal is to help people process the pain and trauma associated with that specific experience, in the context of a safe environment. The pain and torment indicate what we are dealing with—pain gives great insight. We allow them to express any hurt or emotional struggle associated with the memory from the past because this opens the door for release.

Once the memory is on the table, the healing process centers on letting that memory go. Releasing a memory involves focusing either on a person from the past event or the trauma of that experience, and may require forgiving someone or admitting a secret. All of this is done in the context of the grace of God, meaning Jesus paid the price to release the pain. We allow for plenty of expression and insight coming from ministry recipients. This lets them be in control of themselves and their boundaries regarding expression. The flow of the ministry session is kept in prayer, and sensitivity to the Holy Spirit is exercised throughout the session.

The goal is to work through the pain. I find that this is when relying on the Holy Spirit is very helpful. He guides and reveals things that must be faced and released. This step may lead to forgiveness, weeping, praying for deliverance, or a gentle physical embrace, all of which enable the person to be set free from the pain of the memory and trauma surrounding the event.

Many times ungodly beliefs and difficult emotions surface during a ministry session. That is expected. Time is spent correcting false beliefs by reassuring the ministry recipient that this is a time of healing and by enabling them to see the goodness of God's mercy. A time for teaching and imparting truth is necessary too. This allows the minister to give feedback and insight regarding God's Word and the reality of His presence. The minister can become the vehicle for truth and realignment of a person's soul. The hope is that the wounded soul receives the truth and is set free from the pain of the tormenting memory.

This procedure is not foolproof, but when all parties are sensitive to the Holy Spirit's leading, there is the potential for much fruit. The ministry processes provide a path for healing, but the wounded soul must at some point come before God and receive His personal touch in order to be made fully whole. Exchanging the entrenched hurt in the soul with the grace and mercy of Christ is what inner healing and ministry to the memories are all about.

One word of caution: the ministry of inner healing and memory work has some potential pitfalls. There are dangerous things that we can practice that may open us up to ungodly forces or further injury. Remember, never go digging for anything that isn't there. Fabricating memories or past incidences that are not there defeats the process. The goal is to unload a burden, not pick one up. If things are buried, God will bring them to your remembrance when He knows you are ready to deal with them. The soul seems to store things in layers, and each layer involves memories. Those memories are powerful because they continue to control and influence us. We are looking to release the power of whatever binds us, not fabricate it. Most of us have plenty of authentic issues brewing in our souls to work through without adding made-up ingredients to the pot.

Listen, Wait, Obey, and Stand

God has a way of communicating with us that can make this process of inner healing unfold, but we must know how to hear His voice for it to be effective. I call it listening prayer, which is something that I have practiced for years. Learning to hear God's voice provides incredible strength and guidance during the healing process. Basically, we come before God and He speaks to us. Some believe that coming before God is like Dorothy and her bewildered friends coming before the Great Oz in The Wizard of Oz movie. It scares the "waddin" out of us (as my grandmother used to say). Nothing could be further from the truth.

God wants us to know Him, and a big part of that is learning to hear His voice. I received insight regarding this process about fifteen years ago. I believe God gave me four words—listen, wait, obey, and stand—that encompass the active process of hearing God and appropriating His Word into our lives. It is not enough to hear only; we must do, or take action on, the Word.

To listen is simply to receive the words or sounds of another. God has a way of communicating, and for our healing to be complete, we need to hear His words and receive them into our heart. Jesus described this process to the Samaritan woman at the well (John 4:6–26). He told her that God talks to us through spirit and truth. He communicates by spirit because He is Spirit. The words of His Spirit come to us in our hearts. We hear them deep in our being, and they translate to our minds in sentences (usually little, short ones) that we know we could not produce. Often they are profound in nature, declaring who we are or who God is in our lives. Hearing these words in our spirit produces great healing because God's voice silences the voices of pain and fear. No one's voice is more piercing than God's. It cuts to the heart and produces life.

I encourage you to sit quietly before God (in His presence) and listen for His voice (in your heart). Then spend time journaling your thoughts and researching the words you received. Look them up in scripture. This confirms whether they are from God or not. If there are hurts or needs in your life, take those before God, and allow Him to speak to you about them.

The *renewal of the mind* is another critical step to inner healing that is connected to hearing God's voice. For many years I thought memorizing scripture was the key to the renewed mind, so I toiled for hours memorizing verses of the Bible. However, I have come to realize that the healing of a wounded soul requires a much deeper work in the mind. It is the *application* of the Word of God that engrains it into our minds, not just the *memorization* of it. For instance, a football coach can draw plays on a chalkboard and get the concept of the plays into the minds of his players. Yet the concepts are not real to them until they actually run the plays on the field during practice. In the same way, when you act on the Word of God, it becomes real to you; then your mind is transformed. Let's look at an example using fear.

Thoughts of fear are a hindrance to the healing process. I struggled with deep fear when I was sick. The cycle started with the thought that the pain in my body would not go away. The pain was real, and it reinforced the strength of the thoughts of fear. I discovered that I had to recondition my mind with a deeper reality. I used scriptures like 2 Timothy 1:7, "God has not given us a spirit of fear," worked it into my mind, and then did something to activate it. I would read it aloud, meditate on it, and then try to practice it throughout the day. Instead of sitting around and wallowing in my fear, I would call a friend and speak in faith about my struggles, confess out loud the healing of the Lord, eat something healthy (even though I was having a hard time digesting anything), and go for a walk and think about the times that God had already met my needs. All of these actions empowered me to believe, and they still do. Each time I act on God's Word, it sharpens my mind and renews it.

One reason renewing the mind is critical is that it enables us to discern where our thoughts are coming from. Discernment is a gift of the Spirit that gives us a sensitivity to discriminate between good and evil, and gives a keen sense of distinction of the differences. The gift is vital because it helps us recognize the source of our thoughts and urgings. We receive information in our minds from three very different sources: God, ourselves (the flesh), and Satan. Just because beliefs are housed in our soul does not mean they are all from us. Sometimes we buy into a line of thinking because it has been there for so long, and we never discern if it is good or evil.

If these ungodly beliefs overpower our thoughts and our will to make godly choices, we may need to ask for further ministry in deliverance or healing. The key to remember is that God's voice always brings light, which leads to peace, and the devil's voice always brings darkness, which leads to confusion. Our voice is important because ultimately we must agree or disagree with what we are hearing.

Healing is promoted by aiding the body with positive, Bible-based thinking; emotional crises and fear-based thinking exhaust the body and promote sickness. The old "stinking thinking" that says, "Nothing good is going to happen to me," must go. It must literally die. Put away thinking that supports death and exchange it with thinking that supports life. What's really interesting is the paradoxical change that takes place—as we die to our will and our way, new life forms.

Jesus spoke this truth when He said that if a grain of wheat falls to the ground and dies, it will reproduce life (John 12:24). The same principle applies to our soul. As we die to self and fill up on the Word, daily, new life forms. His Word produces new growth on the inside of us.

Out with the Old, In with the New

Over the course of our lives we obtain a reputation, sometimes being labeled as the bad guy (girl) and other times as the good guy (girl). Stereotypes such as these can form our self-image—the way we view ourselves, the way we interact with others, and how we think God views us. I have noticed that the more freedom I've gained in Christ, the more I have changed in these areas. In fact, my self-image is completely different now from what it was when I first started this process thirty years ago.

Intense ministry brings to the surface the "real you." It gives you an opportunity to come to acceptance with your rough edges and empowers you to live above what was said about you in the past. This is good. The Bible says that all of creation awaits the sons of men coming into their purpose and position in life (Rom. 8:19). The person God intends for you to be is the one who is validated during the ministry process. This real you is the one God is calling forward to separate from the past. I want to live in glory. Notice I did not say I live to "be glorified." *Glory* is that bright beam that reflects off of metal as the sun radiates on it. I want to reflect God's glory in that way, so that every hurt in my life (I hope) will be turned into an offering for His honor.

We must learn to separate ourselves from the false self, the one appointed by Satan, our adversary, and embrace the one appointed by God, our Creator. This process is one of agreement: I learn to walk in agreement with who God says I am, and I fall out of agreement with who the accuser says I am. I learn to fall into my Father's arms, and as I stare into the His face (by looking at His Word), I see the true me. His Word for me becomes the person He created me to be.

We hinder the move of God's Spirit in our lives by not obeying His Word, and we create problems for ourselves. For instance, the Word tells us to forgive others. The reason we must forgive is that blaming others for our hurt and wishing revenge complicates the healing process. Until we release others (through forgiveness), we are trapped by our own bitterness toward those who hurt us. The blame game turns into a hypocritical standard because we do not extend to them what we expect the Lord to do for us. We pronounce judgment on our brothers but often expect God to treat us with tender, loving care. If we want God's Word to produce supernatural results in our lives, we have a responsibility to come into agreement with it in this area as well as all others. Obedience is willful submission. It is our responsibility to agree with God's Word by yielding to it. The power of agreement unlocks the door to transformation.

I remember standing on the lawn of my parents' home after a brief visit with them several years ago. The visit came after a seven-year silence. It was the kind of situation where you know that things should be different, but they're not. That weekend was the first time my parents had ever laid eyes on my children. They had never met my kids before because of the separation between us that was much at their request. And even then, the door was only open because we were in town for a class reunion.

I went to visit them, fearing the situation would be sensitive, but the Lord gave me instructions to pull back and allow healing to surface. The weekend turned out to be a sweet and precious time together. During the visit I asked the Lord for an opportunity to seal the weekend on a good note, and He answered my prayer. I had an opportunity to look into my father's eyes, which were riddled with the pain of a hard life, and speak these words (they literally flew out of my mouth): "I am so proud to be your son," to which he replied that he was proud to be my father. Encouraged by this interaction, I went further and said, "I have always loved you, Dad," and he said, "I love you too, son." Those words set in motion a new era in my thinking—I began to view my life and the history of my childhood in a new light. As a result, my relationship with my parents began to be transformed, a process that could not have happened, had I remained bitter toward my father.

I find that we often work hard at being godly, yet we fail miserably because we do not come into agreement with God's Word. Perhaps an important question to ask ourselves is, "Is this really working for me?" In other words, "Is my belief system bringing me into God's peace and purpose?" If the answer is no, then the main reason why our set of beliefs may not be working for us is that God doesn't bless things that grow in darkness. If we expect to walk in the blessings of God and experience scriptural freedom and wholeness, we must live in the light of His presence and His Word. God does not approve of sin or compromise, even if everyone else is doing it.

The Front Door to Denial

The resistance to change in moments of suffering is found in one thing—pride. Pride is the front door to denial. The defense systems we create to prevent modifications of our lifestyle should be packaged and sold to the military and used for strategic warfare. We become professionals when it comes to telling others how to run their lives, but we flop around like fish out of water when making application of our own message. We can preach it, but we find walking it out to be a challenge. Why? The reason is, we do not yield and come into agreement with the Word of God—what we profess to believe on the outside is not what we really believe on the inside. Nevertheless, we hold pride up as a shield because we are afraid.

There are no good reasons to hide behind pride. Pride destroys us. Pride is false security in our abilities, which always fall short. We let pride control us because we do not know God's love in terms of unconditional acceptance. However, it is the deep "knowing" that we have His approval that will give us the foundation we need for change. If we never grasp this principle of unconditional love, we will continue to scurry about, looking for self-justification out of fear and pride. There is no self-justification for wanting our own way in God's economy. Our recognition of this truth will promote trust and confidence in our only hope—the justification of God through the atonement of Jesus Christ.

I know this is a tough message, but remember, it comes from my experience of crawling through the trenches and finding great freedom on the other side of my darkness. The light at the end of this tunnel is the goodness of God.

The bottom line is that if we have emotional wounds, they will block the healing process and hinder growth. Not only will they distort our perception of God, self, and others, but the hurts we carry in life will prevent us from receiving the goodness of God. Can you see why releasing those burdens is so important?

This may be surprising, but the toughest step of the process is allowing God to touch us where we hurt. Most people experience a form of emotional trauma at some point in life. Many experience this during childhood, while for others the injury to the heart comes as adults. Nevertheless, if we have been hurt and we carry it in our hearts, we can be healed of our wounds. God desires to hold us by the hand and walk it out with us, if we will let Him.

The good news is that if we cry out to God in our pain, He will meet us, deliver us, heal us, and restore us to our proper place within the family of God. That is His promise, and He is faithful to His Word. There is no doubting His position.

For me, recognizing my significance in God gives me great joy. I now view life as a gift. When a person comes close to losing his life and is blessed to get it back, as I was, this realization permeates his every waking hour: I died only to learn how to live. That is freedom—no more cutting and pasting my achievements together, hoping for recognition. I am eating at the table of my heavenly Father and sharing the benefits with a lost and dying world. That is a belief to build your life on!

Prayer:

> *Dear heavenly Father, I yield to You. You alone are God; there is no other. I need You. I desperately need You. I cannot live without Your embrace.*
>
> *I ask You to pull me close to Your chest and hold me close to Your heart. Reveal to me any and all wounds in me that are yet to be healed, anything that needs to be transformed by Your touch. Touch me with Your great right hand. Deliver me from the wounds of my childhood, youth, and even adulthood. Take away my sorrows and mend my broken heart. Release the burden*

of my inner pain and create a clean, strong heart within my soul. Repair my broken will, which has been turned inward. Give me hope for healing. Deliver me from myself.

Thank You for meeting me according to Your Word. You are always faithful, and I deeply love You and honor You, Father. I pray in the name of Your Son, Jesus. Amen.

CHAPTER 9

THE MORE
EXCELLENT WAY

The Divine Exchange

All the evil due, by justice, to come to us came on Jesus, so that all the good due to Jesus, earned by His sinless obedience, might be made available to us.

DEREK PRINCE, *Atonement*[1]

AFTER LYING IN BED FOR MONTHS, MY BODY RACKED with disease, I began to crave life. I hungered for something divine. Mentally exhausted from trying to figure out my future and drained of all hope of ever being healed, my cry became, "Would someone please show me God?" I was beaten down by doctors and their dismal prognoses, worn-out from listening to unbelieving Christians who encouraged me to just hang in there, and frazzled by the shadow of death that loomed over me. I needed to meet with God. The good news is He heard my cry.

God met me in my misery. He did not leave me rejected and forsaken in my mess. The Creator of the universe had mercy on me and never gave up on me. He believed that I would make it and that I would overcome. He took me by the hand and led me to a place in Him—a place of safety, healing, and restoration.

Are you hungry for an appointment with God? He's waiting to meet you too.

Sometimes when we hear testimonies of people overcoming difficult situations, we doubt their sincerity. But I am not seeking to pull the wool over your eyes in this book. I have communicated an authentic version of what transpired in my life. Each step of the way, God provided direction and people to help me discover the truth and the unchanging power of the gospel message of Jesus Christ. He has never failed me, and I know He won't fail you either.

When we are suffering for any reason, we need an impartation from God. We need to receive His divine touch. We do not need human reason or sympathy. The words of people may comfort for a moment, but in the long run, they only prevent healing. Our sole hope is a supernatural contact with the living God. Think about the woman in the Bible who had an issue of blood for twelve years. What did she say when she heard that Jesus was nearby? She told herself, "If I can only touch the hem of His garment, I will be made whole;" and when she touched it, she was healed (Matt. 9:20–21). No substitute will do. Only the impartation, the insertion of divine reality, will bring healing and restoration.

God has made the restoration of mankind possible through the life, death, and resurrection of His Son, Jesus Christ. All other remedies play second fiddle. The intention of God is to bring full-scale restoration to the present condition of man, and He planned and prepared a course of events to unveil this mystery at the proper time. He knew that mankind could not save, heal, deliver, or restore itself, so the Savior of the world came to bring complete atonement for the separation that exists between God and man (Titus 3:4–5). This message is still the same today, and it is still quite relevant as well—especially when we consider the present condition in which many of God's people are living.

More Than Eternal Salvation

Most of my Christian life I was taught that Christ died for my sins. How amazing! He provided *atonement*, or *justification*, for my sinful position. These lofty words mean that He paid the price for the punishment I deserve, and His sacrifice provides forgiveness from my sins and gives me a place in heaven for all eternity. Yet, as I discovered, there is so much more to the process than the concern about eternity.

The saving act of Christ, the Messiah, provides restoration for our current condition, whether it's physical disease and malady, emotional pain, mental confusion, or a host of other agonizing positions caused by our separation from God. Yes, Christ endured all the evil due us so that we could receive all the good due Him. Not only did Jesus purchase our right to eternal salvation, but also He provided the reality that I can overcome evil and suffering in this life.

The salvation plan that the prophets of the Old Testament saw in the future for God's people included deliverance, healing, and eternity with God. Their vision for us was not limited to a down payment for a possible seat in heaven someday. It guaranteed our protection, healing, and complete restoration. We just saw that the woman with the issue of blood claimed that if she could touch the hem of Christ's garment, she would be made "whole." This wholeness is a translation of the Greek word *sozo*, which means "to be *saved*," and that includes healing.[2] Jesus looked at her and said, "Your faith has saved you" (Matt. 9:22). We know that the text indicates that she was instantly healed and delivered from the infirmity she had suffered with for many years.

If we ignore the full package Christ offers us, we miss out on the benefits of salvation that are promised to us *in this life*. The blessings are for the present. Have you ever been told at Christmastime that you have to wait to open a present? That's how some believers view what God offers us through His Son. Yet the gospel provisions are ours for receiving today. They are not to be set on the shelf and used like the dishes in the china cabinet that are for looks only. Get them down out of the cupboard and slap some goodies on them and enjoy using them. The goodness of God is for you right now.

A Life-or-Death Bond

The biblical covenant of God is an agreement He made with us. He initiated the union, and so it is founded upon His terms. We were doomed to destruction because of our sin and the lordship of our new master, Satan (who was given the title deed to the earth when Adam fell in the garden). A covenant in God's eyes is an eternal commitment that is founded as the result of the shedding of blood. For that reason, it is a life-or-death contract. The blood covenant between God and mankind was made when His Son, Jesus, shed His blood on the cross for us. There are no halfhearted presuppositions regarding God's commitment to keep His end of the deal. He does not change His posture, regardless of our vacillation to follow through on our dedication to Him.

Therefore, if the covenant of God is a life-or-death bond, then the quality of our life is dependent upon our response to God's initiative to make covenant with us. He pursues us, and we respond to Him. He is the greater party in the covenant, and we need Him. He does not need us to sustain His life. Can you see how the whole thing revolves around God? There is no covenant or salvation without Him. Every aspect of our lives is wrapped up in learning to interact with our Creator. Life flows from Him, and the vehicle for the guidelines of our communication with Him is the blood covenant. It is a treaty between parties, although we cannot dictate the rules of relationship; only God sets up the laws and principles for interaction.

The great thing about our covenant with God is that it's built on His nature and not ours. He is completely invested in our welfare. His imposing of the terms is in our favor. He bases His interaction with us on His lovingkindness, which summarizes His motivation for extending the covenant relationship to us. His lovingkindness is His perfect love, and His movement toward humanity is always founded on this unfailing and embracing love. Not only does He accept us in our weakness and seek to draw us close to Him, but also He offers us an opportunity to be under Him and His protection.

The goal of the blood covenant is that God's nature might become ours. Think about it—God literally wants us to have His genetic code. Here's the reason the blood is so important: the exchanging of blood between two parties causes them to be united on a deep level. This is not a casual thing. Through this exchange, the two parties become one. Remember, Jesus often described His relationship with the Father in terms of being one with Him, and in John 17:11, Jesus prayed that His followers would also become one with the Father. The act of becoming one with God through Christ sets the stage for us to live a life full of blessings.

The Sacrifice

Sin, the collaboration with evil, divides us from God. Our sin cuts us off from receiving from God the resources we need for life. We are governed by a sinful nature, which seeks to find life apart from God and cannot be fulfilled. This inherent nature causes us to live a life filled with lies, which leads to destruction.

The entire first half of the Bible reflects this around-we-go cycle. God rescued the Israelites from their sin and rebellion, they yielded to Him for a season, and then they rebelled against Him again. In turn, God allowed them to experience the fruit of their own devices, but He always ended up pursuing them out of compassion. This scenario perfectly describes our own lives: basically, we blow it—but God is ever faithful to rescue us.

That whole cycle of we-sin-He-saves and we-sin-He-delivers-us is about God's overall plan to redeem us. God is invested in bringing His people into a better way of living, one that is above the fallout of our sinfulness. The word used in the Bible for the process is *atonement*. Though this word may seem archaic in light of man's modern advancements, its relevance is timeless. We cannot cover or erase our own sin. The Old Testament refers to a sacrificial system used to atone for sin, but which yielded little fruit. This practice was based upon a sacrificial system in which the priest placed animals on altars and sacrificed them to remove the sin of a nation for up to one year (See Ex. 29:14). The method was not complete because every year it had to be renewed.

The book of Hebrews in the New Testament provides a clear explanation of why the old way was replaced with a more excellent way (Heb. 7:18–22). The more excellent way provided more than just a covering of sins; it actually removed them or took them away. So the New Covenant, or the new arrangement, gave believers the opportunity to have our sins covered, scattered, and smothered. Our sin, under the new arrangement, is completely removed once and for all—it is gone for good and forgotten by God.

John the Baptist introduced Jesus to the world as the Lamb of God who took away sin (John 1:29), and he was right. Jesus Christ not only covered our sins with His shed blood, He removed them and the consequences they carry with them. Sin is erased for those who are born again if we seek forgiveness and apply the blood of Christ to our sin (remember, we apply the blood by speaking that over ourselves and others).

Jesus was the final high priest in scripture. As High Priest, He offered the sacrifice; and not only that, He Himself was the sacrifice (Heb. 9:25). He placed Himself on the altar and gave His life as payment for our sin. The concept of Jesus as both High Priest and Lamb (sacrifice) is huge because it offers us a number of truths about the nature of God: (1) He takes our sin very seriously, (2) He expects us to be righteous, and (3) the thing He requires He provides (2 Cor. 5:21). All this is done on our behalf through God's goodness.

This holy act of pure righteousness is the essence of what the cross resembles for the modern-day believer. The cross is the center for our faith. We have no salvation, miracles, move of the Spirit, or forgiveness of sin without the finished work of the cross. Upon this one act rests our entire foundation for health. The work of Christ on the cross enables those who follow after Him to live a life of wholeness.

Sin will continue to erode our health unless there is a supernatural way to undo that process—and the gospel message is that process.

Jesus came in the flesh to empower us to overcome the downward spiral of sin and therefore live a new, healthy life. We overcome sin by trusting in the work of Christ who paved the way for us to live a free life. We can now honestly say, "I am free because I am no longer chained to my sinful nature. I now live by the new nature God gave me through believing and following Christ, my Lord. Even my conscience is purged from dead works, or unbelief, which brings death."

This newfound liberty gives me the strength to face the consequences of my sin. I now have a way to work out my problems. God gives me grace to face everything that goes wrong in my life, including the things I cause and the afflictions that others put on me. Even Satan's attack against me now serves to my benefit because the Lord rises up within me, causing me to defeat my foe. This means that now I am being perfected. In other words, this is a perfect work for an imperfect person who is learning to be perfected. The sacrifice of Christ is perfect. It is finished!

Some scoff at this remarkable offer by God, insulting God's goodness by doubting the sacrifice and its worthiness. But unbelief will only leave us in a position of utter destruction. If we reject God's offer and choose not to enter into this wonderful relationship with the Lord, then we condemn ourselves. We cannot expect God to make our bed for us. He provided the healing, deliverance, and salvation, but we must appropriate His work into our lives. I've heard some people say, "I guess if God is going to heal me, He will heal me." No, they have it all wrong. God's work is complete in Christ, but we must act in faith to receive it. Remember, it is like a bank vault full of money. Knowing that the bank vault is full does us no earthly good if we do not take action to draw out the money. We must go after it.

At one point, I heard God say the words, "Come after Me," but it sounded to me like He was saying, "Tackle Me." Those are powerful words to an old football player. Today, I am learning to go for it. In other words, I'm diving into the Word of God each day, and I'm making daily application of the Word in my life, as well.

The Divine Exchange

The *divine exchange* is about learning to surrender the weight of our sin and its consequences through the finished work of the cross. There can be no change, no Pentecost (Acts 2), without Calvary. We must realize that if our lives are overwhelmed by the fruit of our sin, then we are not properly appropriating the finished work of the cross. I sometimes wish I could get out of my car at a busy intersection and ask people if they are truly satisfied with their lives. I know that sounds outrageous, but I believe I could predict the response I would get if I polled people on that question. I'm sure that most would allude to something unfinished or a greater need in their life being unmet. Christians, I find, are no different. Many of us do not know how to move through our suffering with an understanding of how to become victorious over it.

That's why I am calling believers to the table of the divine exchange. It is possible for us to meet with a counselor who actually has answers that will resolve our sufferings. Believe it or not God planned, set up, and perfected a way that gives us all the liberty to resolve our struggles with Him. He invites us to come into His presence, sit before Him, and bring our diseases, our shame, our guilt, our rejection, our pain, our suffering, our misery, our poverty, and any other malady so that we can exchange them for His more excellent way.

The more excellent way is that I get to exchange my disease for health, my shame for glory, my poverty for wealth, and my fear for peace. He takes my bad junk and gives me His perfect gifts. That is a swap meet that is hard to turn down. There is no greater offer. All of my sin and its consequences were placed on Jesus at the cross and, in return, I receive all of the blessings and rights due to Him because of His obedience. That's what the quote at the beginning of this chapter was referring to. Doesn't that sound like an incredible plan? It may sound too good to be true, but I know it is real. My life is a testimony of someone who could not get it right—I could not do things the right way—and yet God turned my life around.

Our Spiritual Legal Rights

Imagine if we were called before the Supreme Court of the land to review our right to our citizenship and sitting on the throne of judgment were the highest authorities of the land, the Supreme Court justices. Though they might appear intimidating, the one thing that would determine whether we were granted the freedom to stay in this country or were deported to another nation under a harsh dictator would be the way we approach them. What would we base our right to citizenship on? The law. The law states that if we were born in this country, we have a legal right to citizenship. It is our birthright. So we would present the high court with a birth certificate issued by the hospital where we were born because it would take a legal document to prove our rights. The judges would review the document and approve our citizenship because we were covered by our birthrights.

Our spiritual heritage is similar. We have legal rights as believers because we have a spiritual birthright. Upon our confession that Jesus Christ is our new Lord, we moved our citizenship from the kingdom of this world to the kingdom of heaven. We changed our residency to belong to God. We are no longer under the rule of the evil tyrant, Satan. He no longer has rights to us. However, he seeks to convince us that we are still his slaves.

That's what happened when slavery was outlawed in this country in the mid-1800s. Many African-American people who had been slaves were convinced they could not leave or they would be killed—and the slave owners were trying to keep them in bondage. This is what the enemy of our soul tries to do to us. He acts as if we are still his servants, but he knows that he does not have legal right to tell us what to do. Nevertheless, if we listen to him, we give him that power. That is why we need to educate ourselves about our spiritual legal rights.

If we do not want to be pushed around by that evil "slave owner," we need to know how to defend ourselves against him. When we start going through the exchange process, he will try to convince us that we are disqualified. But our rights include knowing who we are, because our identity changed when we became born again. We are no longer just a son or daughter of a father born into the devil's slavery. We now have access to the president of the country. Jesus gives us a heritage that says what He possesses and owns, we own. It is ours because He gave it to us.

Paul used the term *heir(s)* in Romans 4 and 8, and again in Galatians 4 to describe our legal right to freedom from the oppression of sin and the law. In these passages, he explains that the law could never save us from sin. *Heir* in his writings speaks of our entitlement to walk in authority as freedmen. As heirs, we have been given the authority to fulfill the law and overcome sin and the powers of darkness. We are heirs of the good things, the blessings of God, because our Lord has presented an acceptable case for our sin.

Jesus is our advocate who makes intercession for us. He is our attorney, taking care of the mess we have made of our lives. This does not mean we have the right to act foolishly and expect Jesus to cover our tracks for us, though. No, our authority is only good if we do our part—obey Him. If we do not live according to the laws He set up, then we must be disciplined and taught how to live.

Exchanging Sin with Righteousness

Isaiah's gospel foretells the whole story of the mission of Jesus Christ. The foundation for Isaiah's prophecy is recorded in the fifty-third chapter. The core issue is the removal of sin; Isaiah centers his message on that subject.

> *All we like sheep have gone astray; we have turned, each one to his own way; and Jehovah has laid on Him the iniquity of us all.*
> ISAIAH 53:6

Here is the ultimate root of all of our problems—sin. We are willfully separated from God because we choose our own way. The stubbornness of our actions produced hardness toward God, and we find ourselves wracked with undeniable consequences for our sin. We get sick, we divorce our mates, we handle our money irresponsibly, we lose our jobs, and we hurt ourselves and others. How are we to fix ourselves? It is impossible; we cannot fix the sin problem. We have tried every imaginable means to fixing it and been unsuccessful. That is why the Son of God came to earth. He came to fix the sin problem.

Isaiah makes it clear that the weight of our sin problem was placed upon Him, the Christ. Later, Paul writes in his letters to the Colossians and Ephesians that Christ redeemed us, which means He bought us back from slavery. He paid the price for our sin with His shed blood, and that price was acceptable to God. Now we may be washed and cleansed from our sin with Jesus' blood and "the washing of water by the Word" (Eph. 5:26).

That does not mean we have to wait until eternity to experience purity. We can have a sense of cleanness or holiness now. We experience the cleansing as we allow God to purge from our lives all worldliness and darkness. As He continues to wash us, the purification truly increases our quality of life. We become better people in the process.

Exchanging Wounds with Healing

Why was the death of Christ so brutal? The only innocent man who ever lived died the cruelest and most agonizing death in history. His crucifixion was brutal, for He took upon His body our physical suffering. Although the physical atonement was not the only focus, it was a significant part of it. Jesus took blows to His body because He knew it would release us from the blows we have taken to our bodies. All the pain inflicted on Him releases us from our suffering.

Isaiah 53:4 says, "Surely He has borne our griefs, and carried our sorrows; yet we esteemed Him stricken, smitten of God, and afflicted." The Hebrew words for *griefs* and *sorrows* are interpreted as "sicknesses"[3] and "physical pains."[4] These two terms include every physical malady known to man. The reality is that without Jesus' sacrifice, we have no hope, especially those of us who suffer with chronic problems.

Peter in his first letter takes this scripture and amplifies it. He says that by the stripes of Christ we "were healed" (1 Peter 2:24). He puts the past atonement work of Christ into the present. He is saying that the work of Christ, which happened in a different era of time, heals us today. Our healing is as final as the fact that our sins are forgiven. The healing atonement of Christ is still valid, if we believe.

If we expect to exchange our infirmity with His provision of health, we must believe that He desires to heal us. We cannot receive healing if we do not believe that God is a healer. If we think that God gave us our disease to teach us a lesson, we will not turn to Him to release us. Regardless of how we contracted the sickness—whether self-induced, an accident, or an unknown cause—we cannot receive healing until we look to God. He is the only healer who seeks to save us in the process.

Healing can occur through various means, including a miracle, recovery over time, a series of healings, or a variety of these methods. Recognize that the mode is not the priority, but the connection to God and experiencing His guidance are the most important elements in the process. It is our responsibility to come to God with our pain. When we receive His direction, we need to act on it and apply it to our life. His Word becomes the seed that begins the growth process for healing; the seed is planted through the spoken Word. We can speak or others can share it with us, but we move forward each day, taking the Word as our medicine.

Healing comes as we exchange the pain of our infirmity for the reality of God's provision for health. James says in his letter that we must act on our beliefs: "As the body without the spirit is dead, so faith without works is dead" (James 2:26). In other words, faith is not faith until it becomes an action. The action follows the principles laid out for us in God's Word. The fact is that action steps make His Word real to us. We meditate on the Word, focus on it, and stand on it by faith, knowing that it supplies our spirit with strength, which trickles down to our body. The body responds to the soul, and healing begins and continues to wholeness.

Exchanging Shame with Glory

We addressed the need and process of emotional or inner healing in a previous chapter, but we're going to look at it here in the context of the divine exchange. This aspect of the exchange process continues the understanding of why and how God heals us in those deep wounds. The shame of our sinfulness is compounded by emotional wounds to the soul. All the dark blows we receive from others damage the soul; they may come from family or foe, but they all injure the heart.

Soulish hurts do not just go away because we grow up. They must be faced and worked through in our lives. Working out these hurts takes place as we bring them to the cross, the safest place in the world to deal with our hurt. The Savior of the cross embraces us and empowers us to overcome everything we need to face.

Crucifixion was looked upon as the most despicable type of death in Jesus' day, yet the writer of Hebrews records that He despised the shame of the cross (Heb. 12:2). This means He moved through the horrific public event of crucifixion with disregard,[5] knowing that it would bring healing and deliverance to those of us who experienced shameful emotional wounds in our lives. What did He choose to disregard? The event of His death involved an open display of His body, His dignity, and His right to privacy, and forced Him to be exposed to public humiliation—Jesus was completely disgraced and shamed before the entire community of His day. How does that affect us? He was unjustly abused so that our blows of abuse could be released.

We release our shame in exchange for His glory. The shame is discharged as we invite the Holy Spirit to work in us and remove the stain of the sinful hurts we received. For that to happen, we must open the door to all secrets and false beliefs we hold as a result of the internal pain we received from those who hurt us. Something else exchanging our shame for His glory means is that we are honored as sons and daughters who are loved by the Father. This takes us from a low, guilt-ridden position to a position of health and wholeness. Receiving His glory means that we become the people we were ordained to be before creation. We find our place of security, and that position—not the guilt of the past—defines our future.

Exchanging Rejection with Acceptance

Acceptance is a critical piece to our welfare as individuals. We need to know that we belong. The push in our culture is to find approval from others, but the truth is, some of us spend a lifetime looking for approval from others and never get it. The acceptance of others is fleeting because they struggle with the same problems we do. So how do we find acceptance?

Acceptance is perfect love. That love comes from those who are able to love (or accept) us for who we are. They reach out to us and embrace us with all of our flaws. They do not walk away from us because they notice a quirk or a struggle in our lives. Rather, they have the ability to look into our heart and believe in us, recognizing that we are imperfect. This kind of love only comes from God. We can experience His perfect love by receiving it from Him and from people such as these who are filled with His Spirit.

In the Old Testament, this type of love is called lovingkindness. I believe the best example of lovingkindness is found in the life and prophecies of Hosea because this prophet was summoned by God to marry a prostitute. Hosea was sent by God into the worst part of town to find this ungodly woman to betroth her. He was instructed to take her as his wife because God was making the illustration to His people (then and now) that He would do the same for them. He would meet them in the low places and take them to be His bride, with all of their sin and shamefulness. Hosea 2:19 says, "I will betroth you to Me forever. Yea, I will betroth you to Me in righteousness, and in judgment, and in lovingkindness, and in mercies." This passage illustrates the heart of God toward His people.

We are God's people when we become born again, and the extension of His grace toward us (His people) is still motivated by His lovingkindness. His covenant love toward His people is sealed with the blood of His own Son. He provided the death of His Son as a demonstration of His unconditional love toward us. The love of God is real because the man Jesus of Nazareth was and is real.

This acceptance is unlike our conditional relationships that we form with each other. We say we are committed to one another, but we flee at the slightest hint of weakness. Most of the time our relationships are one-sided, and we do not experience unconditional love. That is why it is so hard for us to grasp the love of God. His love is perfect and ours is motivated by selfish gain. We put people on trial in our lives. We say, "*If* you do what I want, *then* you may have my approval." But the if/then cycle is a never ending roller coaster of disappointments.

God's way of relating to us is quite different than man's way. He says to us, "I accept you and I want you to know Me according to My perfect love," and He holds us until we know we are loved. He bases each move in the relationship on His lovingkindness. Isaiah 54:6 says, "For Jehovah has called you as a woman forsaken and grieved in spirit, and a wife of youth, when you were rejected, says your God." Likewise, Jesus came to demonstrate the acceptance and love of the Father toward His people.

Jesus was criticized for spending time with low-life people, prostitutes, drunkards, criminals, and others despised by the pious people of His day. Yet where He spent His time indicates that He recognized the weaknesses of people and communicated His acceptance to them. For example, He did not reject the woman caught in adultery after her accusers left the scene (John 8:9–10). However, He did warn her to sin no more (v. 11), a good example of the fact that Jesus accepts the sinner but does not tolerate the sin. He knew that sin (adultery in this case) almost cost her life. He wanted her to be free, not just from rejection but from the bondage of sexual sin as well.

> *He is despised and rejected of men; a Man of sorrows, and acquainted with grief; and as it were a hiding of faces from Him, He being despised, and we esteemed Him not . . . But He was wounded for our transgressions; He was bruised for our iniquities; the chastisement of our peace was on Him.*
>
> ISAIAH 53:3, 5

This clearly indicates that Jesus was rejected so that we would be accepted. All the rejection due to us was put upon Him so that in exchange we might receive all the acceptance that was due the Lord. We receive His blessing in place of our rightful punishment.

This reality brings great healing on the emotional level for those who learn to absorb it. If we have spent our lives striving for approval, we are offered the opportunity to lay down our striving and pick up the real truth—that in Christ we are accepted by God. Romans 5:1 says that we have peace with God because of Christ. We no longer have to chase after others to get it; we simply bring our rejection to God and exchange it for His approval.

His unconditional love in our lives empowers us to embrace others who have been wounded and rejected. We become "real" people who introduce others to the love of God. We can mirror God's love to one another because He first loved us. Surprisingly, I find that the greatest struggle in the church is connected to showing and receiving God's love. It seems elementary, but it is true—we need to learn how to love one another. It will only happen as we learn to receive God's love for ourselves.

Exchanging Poverty with Wealth

If you want to pick a fight in a church, just start talking about how money should be spent. More churches are split over money than anything else. It happens because we know that with money comes power. That power enables us to control the course of events in our lives and churches. Basically, we want to be in control. Paul told Timothy that "the love of money is a root of all evil" (1 Tim. 6:10). This startling fact produces many problems in lives, families, churches, businesses, and all other facets of life.

Does money have a worthy purpose in life? Yes, Solomon said that money answers all things (Eccl. 10:19). I believe this means that money helps us to get things, but it does not help us to get the most important things. What we need to buy in order to live is significant—food, clothing, shelter, transportation, and other material goods that we need to do business and serve our purpose. Yet money cannot buy us significance, purpose, or love and acceptance; these come from God. Money and wealth help us sustain life, but they don't make life secure.

The problem for those who experience poverty is that they expect money to pull them up out of this pit when, in actuality, the poverty pit is about a belief system, not a bank account. Consider the words of Paul to the church at Philippi: "I learned to abound. I learned to be without" (Phil. 4:11–12, my paraphrase). In other words, his security was in knowing that God would take care of him. He may have been afraid of lean times, but he knew that God would meet him according to his needs. His belief system indicates to us that he was leading a life of faith in God.

We often operate in fear regarding our wealth. The symptom of our fear is our debt. Most people have more debt than assets. For many, their debt-to-asset ratio is off the charts because they buy things out of fear and insecurity, hoping to make themselves feel better and to gain a place of importance in the world. This vicious cycle grows until it becomes out of control, and they no longer can take the stress. The debt can then lead to bankruptcy, divorce, and a host of other problems.

Income has nothing to do with a poverty mentality because poverty thinking is rooted in fear. We can earn millions or pennies and have a poverty spirit. The motivation driving us to spend money is the key. If we just have to have something, that is false security and immature. It is not what Christ taught His disciples on the Sermon on the Mount. Matthew 6:33 says, "Seek first the kingdom of God and His righteousness; and all these things shall be added to you." This tells me that if I want security regarding my finances, I must first trust God and put my energy into knowing His provision before I look to the things of this world to make me feel secure.

I believe that many of us come from families who have a poverty mentality. They taught us that we do not deserve nice things. The family I grew up in valued hard work as the only means to gaining wealth. There is nothing wrong with hard work, but all the blessings we have come because of the goodness of God, not by the work of our hands. Some people teach us how to manipulate the system to gain security. This leads to problems because we live a life of rebellion if we are cheating others to get our needs met. Whatever the mentality or set of values that we are taught, there is a need to exchange poverty thinking with God's favor.

> *For you know the grace of our Lord Jesus Christ, that, though He was rich, for your sakes He became poor, in order that you might be made rich through His poverty.*
>
> 2 CORINTHIANS 8:9

This verse means that we exchange our poverty for an inheritance of great wealth that includes material blessings and well-being. I find that we have lost sight of moderation in this country. We live in a super-sized world with limitless appetites for more. This does not take away from God's blessings, because He wants us to know security and abundance so that we are able to bless others. I believe God's design for wealth is that we become givers above being takers. We do not have to have everything we want, but if our focus becomes helping others, we graduate into God's economy and way of doing things.

The beginning of this exchange starts with recognizing the false beliefs we have about money. We must lay down our sinful thinking that says money makes us valuable. No, we are valuable because God is our Father and we share His wealth. Laying down the false beliefs also means taking action to unload debt. That includes actual debt as well as the mentality that produces debt. God does not want us to be debtors. Solomon said that the borrower is subject to the lender (Prov. 22:7). If that is the case, we have many lords who rule our lives. That is evident in the fact that we have too much debt, but the exchange process includes releasing the debt and the debtors who owe us.

The moment we put God's principles into action, He opens the door for us to receive His abundance. I know from personal experience that God takes better care of us than we could ever do for ourselves. We cannot beat God's plan for wealth. His Word says in the prophecy of Malachi that if we yield our firstfruits to Him, then He will pour out blessings on us (Mal. 3:10). This is His offer to us, and I believe His plan works better than anything the power thinkers on Wall Street could ever devise.

The Blessings of Trust

God provided for both the forgiveness of my sin and the consequences brought on by my sinful condition. The reason I find that so many people are uncomfortable with discussing sin is that they fear there is no remedy for their plight. I, in turn, want to yell, "Jesus Christ came as a real man into the real world to meet you in your real suffering! He is the only answer for the world today!"

The authority of Christ authenticates His work. He was given authority here on earth by the Father to complete the covenant between God and humanity. That means His work brought closure and satisfaction to the deal between God and man, as His shed blood sealed the deal. He fulfilled all the requirements set by the Father to eliminate the power of sin over us. He was perfect and without sin and obeyed the Father until His last breath. Therefore, His actions bring empowerment to His followers.

John, one of His disciples, recorded a very interesting scenario regarding the requirements of the followers of Christ. In John 6:28, the people following Christ had been with Him for some time and had seen His miracles and heard His teachings. Then they posed this question, "What shall we do that we might work the works of God?" (v. 28). That's what we all want to know today, "How do I become a player in this game? What must I do to experience the benefits of God?" Christ's answer was so powerful. He said that in order to work the works of God you must *believe* on the One He sent (v. 29).

To believe on Him is to entrust your whole life to Him. Since the Fall in the Garden of Eden, the ongoing struggle of the human heart has been to totally trust God. Even in this situation with these people who were following Christ in John 6, no sooner did He say that than they tried to get Him to qualify Himself by showing them miracles. This occurred on the heels of Jesus miraculously feeding the five thousand (John 6:2–13). Sometimes I believe we are blind to seeing God because we want to create Him in our own image—"You do it my way, God, then I will trust You."

If we are going to see the works of God, we must trust Him for who He is. Trust starts with believing His Word. We either believe the truth as it is written, or we will spend our lives in doubt and confusion. Many fall away because they will only believe what makes them feel good. Christ did not shed His blood because it felt good. He did it as a demonstration of His love for us.

Lifeline to a New You

The atonement of Christ is about the divine exchange that God Almighty has made available to every willing soul. I don't know about you, but the high-minded discussion about why and how God made this exchange always seems to lose me. I need to have it broken down for me in simple terms, so I'm going to do the same for you.

The divine exchange is the genius of God. He offers us a lifeline to lift us out of the pit of our lives because He understands our condition, our suffering and pain, and out of a heart of compassion wants to rescue us. This offering is based upon His goodness and unconditional love. Unlike human love, God is unlimited in His mercy and acceptance of us, and He longs to hold us in His embrace until we are restored. This proposal comes to us with an invitation, not a demand.

The heavenly Father not only wants to rescue us from self-destruction, He also wants to equip us to become great overcomers. He engages us and compels us along the race of life, knowing His plans and purposes for us are excellent.

His love may be unconditional, but the offer is not. There are terms that we must recognize before we accept it. He expects, in return, that we lay down our whole life. God's exchange involves old life for new life. This covenant between us is a relationship, a bond, based on His provision and our cooperation. God said that He will impart life to us, but in return He expects us to yield our life to Him. In essence, we are to make a commitment to deny our right to run our own life. We are to follow Him, and we will then receive our just reward for doing so.

This arrangement is awesome. We get to be a partaker, as Peter put it, of divine nature (2 Peter 1:4). The God-man connection becomes real as we daily lay down our rights and, as a replacement, receive God's power to live a supernatural life. The real God, Christ in the flesh, gives us power to move beyond the basic humanistic perspective of reward and punishment. He fills our life with purpose. The living God uses us to impart life to a dying world. Along the way we get to dance with Him, be connected to Him, rejoice with our family and friends about Him . . . and live!

We get to live because of His presence in our life. Every weakness in our life is turned into strength because we have this *real* connection with Him. When we fall prey to evil, we run to Him. When we discover something shocking about the world, we run to Him. When our children look into our face and see His glory, we run to Him. When we get to be intimate with our wife (husband) or spend time with other loved ones, we run to Him. He is in us and we are in Him, and that's worth running into His arms. This life is good, not because it is a life based on pretense but because it is a life based on the truth.

Let me break it down a little more: You do not have to strive to find His approval; you already have it by receiving Christ. You do not have to become religious in order to serve Him; He will take you as you are because of Christ. You do not have to become perfect in order to be justified; you already have been made just and righteous because of Christ. You do not have to worry about having your needs met; they are already met in Christ. You do not have to fear evil; He has already overcome it through Christ. You do not have to suffer from the oppression of guilt and shame anymore; Christ took all of that upon His body as He hung on the cross. You do not have to work up the strength to win your personal battles with sin, sickness, and human weakness; Christ has already made it possible to overcome even death because He was resurrected from the grave.

There is not one thing that is impossible for those who choose to exchange their life with Christ's. I am still learning to apply this principle to my own life as I continue to break free from all that separates me from my spiritual birthright. The whole process of the gospel is about this divine exchange.

If you can get this, it can transform your life and make it much easier. Yet, as we have discussed all throughout this book, the death of Christ and His resurrection are meaningless if we do not first receive new life for ourselves and then apply the kingdom principles to our lives. It is like inheriting millions of dollars from some unknown relative. If I do not draw the money out of the bank and use it, then it is worthless. But when I go to the bank, take out cash, and spend it, then it has power. The same applies for the broken body and shed blood of Jesus. It must be applied to our lives. I'm so glad that I *finally* learned this principle.

I had spent almost thirty years in the church and yet never really knew my authority in Christ. For that matter, I had little real understanding of my identity as a born-again, Spirit-filled believer in Jesus. I believed He died for my sins. I believed the Holy Spirit gave power to believers to do the works of Christ. I knew I had eternal security. I believed the Bible from cover to cover. But I did not know who I was in relation to the atoning sacrifice of Jesus. I conceived that I was a worker and a son in the family of God, but I struggled to appropriate His authority to overcome evil and my struggles with sin.

The apostle Paul used the terminology over and over in his writings that he was "in Christ." That phrase was a foreign concept to me. I was unsure of what it meant—the teaching was unclear. How could I, a sinful being, have Christ in me? That made little sense. Finally, it became real to me when I picked up a copy of the book *Atonement* by well-known author and Bible teacher Derek Prince. He taught that the atonement of Christ was God's provision for mankind's sinful condition.

After I read his book, the concept "in Christ" started to click. Because God realized that we could never clean up ourselves (I had surely realized that about myself), He set up a covenant with His people to establish a real and abiding relationship with Him. This covenant involved a bond between two parties that was sealed by the shedding of blood. As we saw earlier, the old covenant was sealed by the shedding of animal's blood (under the old Law), the new or more improved covenant was based upon the shedding of the blood of Christ—the establishment of a new covenant.

Basically, at the cross Christ endured all the evil due to us and, in turn, made available to us all the good due Him. I made that statement before, but are you starting to get it now? We are under the blessing of Christ, in perfect union with Him. Everything Christ obtained for us through His life, death, and resurrection is ours. We do not have to live under the bondage of sin, which includes rejection, bitterness, fear, envy, jealousy, hatred, addiction, sickness, or any other fruit of sinful core beliefs, damaged emotions, broken hearts, curses, or evil spirits invading our lives.

This concept of freedom became real to me when I received the revelation that Christ my Messiah made a way for me that I could not make for myself. This is my reality. God the Father sent His Son, a real man, into the real earth, at a critical point in the history of mankind, to meet us in our real sufferings. That act of grace was not cheap. It required the offering and obedience of the most valuable life in the history of the world.

It's Time to Get Real

I remember when I went to see my doctor and she gave me a clean bill of health. What a feeling of exhilaration! I was free. I was healed. I was whole. I knew God's Word was true. I was a new man. My whole perception of life was completely different. Before, it was about what I could do, what hill I could climb. Not anymore. After I was healed it was about operating in peace and in cooperation. I was broken in the right place, and I was ready to advance God's kingdom, not my own.

Another important change I experienced was that I had a totally different sense about relationships. I was able to connect and have intimacy with my wife. I respected her for standing with me through the crisis and believing for our lives to get better. Her strength was so crucial for me. She had experienced deliverance from depression and she was a different woman—her parenting of the children had totally changed and she blossomed into a great woman of God.

I noticed, too, that my affection for my children doubled. I never knew how much love a parent could have for a child until I almost lost my opportunity to be a parent. I loved holding them and speaking softly to them. I saw them as gifts from God, not just liabilities I was responsible for. Before, my fear had been passed to them; now my peace was being passed to them instead. My life was transformed, and our family was restored because of it.

I have found that since this season in my life, I have become more aware of the presence of God. He is so real to me now—He is present with me, and I know His touch on the inside of me. I am aware when I am allowing my heart to get cloudy, and I want to resolve my sin issues before the sun goes down. Running to my heavenly Father with open arms is a daily pleasure, not a chore. I find His comforting counsel so sweet and passionate. I would not trade all the worldly success I could ever acquire for His abiding peace in my heart and in my life.

That is my story. For now, I am learning more each day to live "from" Him. I receive new revelation and insight all the time. Often I find it to be so simple. Even when I get back into times of striving and forcing life, He gently leads me back to life that is anchored in the unforced rhythm of His grace. I cherish this process. I am thankful for what I have lost and for what I gained.

When I find myself evaluating my efforts, it is not about how many stars I have collected or how powerful I have become or even how devout my service is. It is about surrendering my life to my Creator and Savior in such a way that He enables me to lock arms with the sick, the dying, the hurting, and the lost, and help them across the finish line, for His glory. That, to me, is the ultimate purpose of a transformed life.

ENDNOTES

Chapter 2

1. Adam Clarke, *Adam Clarke Commentary*, available from http://www
.studylight.org/com/acc/view.cgi?book=joh&chapter=020, s.v. "Receive ye
the Holy Ghost," John 20:22.

2. *John Gill's Exposition of the Entire Bible*, available from http://www
.studylight.org/com/geb/view.cgi?book=joh&chapter=020&verse=022, s.v.
"And saith unto them, receive ye the Holy Ghost," John 20:22.

Chapter 3

1. C.S. Lewis, *The Screwtape Letters* (HarperSanFrancisco; New Ed
edition, 2001).

Chapter 6

1. Albert Barnes, *Albert Barnes' Notes on the Bible*, available from http://
www.studylight.org/com/bnn/view.cgi?book=eph&chapter=006, s.v. "Verse
14. Of Righteousness," Ephesians 6.

2. Based on information from *The People's New Testament*, available from
http://bible.crosswalk.com/Commentaries/PeoplesNewTestament/pnt
.cgi?book=eph&chapter=006, s.v. "14–16," Ephesians 6.

3. *Vincent's Word Studies*, available from http://www.godrules.net/library/
vincent/vincenteph6.htm, s.v. "Chapter VI, 15."

4. Ibid.

5. Based on information from *John Gill's Exposition of the Entire Bible*, available from http://eword.gospelcom.net/comments/ephesians/gill/ephesians6.htm, s.v. "Ephesians 6, Verse 15."

6. *The People's New Testament*, available from http://bible.crosswalk.com/Commentaries/PeoplesNewTestament/pnt.cgi?book=eph&chapter=006, s.v. "17. Take the helmet of salvation," Ephesians 6.

7. Based on information from Adam Clarke, available from http://www.studylight.org/com/acc/view.cgi?book=eph&chapter=006, s.v. "Verse 18. Praying Always," Ephesians 6:18.

8. Albert Barnes, available from http://studylight.org/com/bnn/view.cgi?book=eph&chapter=006, s.v. "Verse 18. Praying Always," Ephesians 6:18.

Chapter 7

1. A. R. Fausset, *Commentary Critical and Explanatory on the Whole Bible*, "Commentary on Galatians 3," available from <http://bible.crosswalk.com/Commentaries/JamiesonFaussetBrown/jfb.cgi?book=ga&chapter=003>.

2. Based on information from the U.S. Department of Energy's "Ask a Scientist" Web site, Molecular Biology Archive, available from http://www.newton.dep.anl.gov/askasci/mole00/mole00338.htm, s.v. "Blood and Fetal Development."

3. This death angel was "a good . . . angel . . . even such a one as was employed in destroying the whole host of the Assyrians in one night (2 Kings 19:35) and answers better in the antitype or emblem to the justice of God taking vengeance on ungodly sinners, when it is not suffered to do the saints any harm." John Gill, available from http://eword.gospelcom.net/comments/exodus/gill/exodus12.htm, s.v. "Verse 23," Exodus 12:23.

Chapter 8

1. Thayer and Smith, *The KJV New Testament Greek Lexicon*, "Greek Lexicon entry for Teknon," available from http://www.biblestudytools.net/Lexicons/Greek/grk.cgi?number=5043&version=kjv, s.v. "sons," John 1:12 (KJV).

2. Based on information from Brown, Driver, Briggs and Gesenius, *The KJV Old Testament Hebrew Lexicon,* "Hebrew Lexicon entry for Y@hovah," available from http://www.biblestudytools.net/Lexicons/Hebrew/heb.cgi?number=3068&version=kjv, s.v. "LORD"; and "Hebrew Lexicon entry for Rapha," available from http://www.biblestudytools.net/Lexicons/Hebrew/heb.cgi?number=7495&version=kjv, s.v. "healeth," Exodus 15:26.

Chapter 9

1. Derek Prince, *Atonement: Your Appointment with God* (Grand Rapids, MI: Chosen Books, 2000), p. 37.

2. Based on information from Thayer and Smith, *The KJV New Testament Greek Lexicon*, "Greek Lexicon entry for Sozo," available from http://www.biblestudytools.net/Lexicons/Greek/grk.cgi?number=4982&version=kjv, s.v. "whole," Matthew 9:21.

3. Brown, Driver, Briggs and Gesenius, "Hebrew Lexicon entry for Choliy," available from http://www.biblestudytools.net/Lexicons/Hebrew/heb.cgi?number=2483&version=kjv, s.v. "griefs," Isaiah 54:4.

4. Ibid., "Hebrew Lexicon entry for Mak'ob," available from http://www.biblestudytools.net/Lexicons/Hebrew/heb.cgi?number=4341&version=kjv, s.v. "sorrows," Isaiah 54:4.

5. Based on information from Albert Barnes, "Commentary on Hebrews 12," available from http://www.studylight.org/com/bnn/view.cgi?book=heb&chapter=012, s.v. "Verse 2; Despising the Shame."